Prostatic Hyperplasia

New Developments in Biosciences 5

Walter de Gruyter
Berlin · New York 1989

Prostatic Hyperplasia

Etiology, Surgical and Conservative Management

Editors
R. Ackermann · F. H. Schröder

Walter de Gruyter
Berlin · New York 1989

Editors

R. Ackermann, M.D.
Professor and Chairman
Department of Urology
University of Düsseldorf
Medical School
Moorenstr. 5
D-4000 Düsseldorf
F.R. Germany

F. H. Schröder, M.D.
Professor and Chairman
Department of Urology
Erasmus University Rotterdam
P.O. Box 1700
NL-3000 DR Rotterdam
The Netherlands

Deutsche Bibliothek Cataloging-in-Publication Data

Prostatic hyperplasia : etiology, surgical and conservative management ; [this monograph is dedicated to Professor Dr. H. G. W. Frohmüller on the occasion of his sixtieth anniversary] / ed. R. Ackermann ; F. H. Schröder. - Berlin ; New York : de Gruyter, 1989

(New developments in biosciences ; 5)
ISBN 3-11-011865-3 (Berlin)
ISBN 0-89925-528-0 (New York)

NE: Ackermann, Rolf [Hrsg.]; Frohmüller, Hubert G. W.: Festschrift; GT

Library of Congress Cataloging-in-Publication Data

Prostatic hyperplasia : etiology, surgical and conservative management / editors, R. Ackermann, F. H. Schröder.
– (New developments in biosciences : 5)
Includes bibliographies.
ISBN 0-89925-528-0
1. Prostate – Hypertrophy. 2. Prostate – Hypertrophy – Surgery.
I. Ackermann, R. (Rolf), 1941– · II. Schröder, F. H. · III. Series.
[DNLM: 1. Prostatic Hypertrophy. 2. Prostatic Neoplasms.
W3 NE865 v. 5 / WJ 752 P9668]
RC899.P68 1989
616.6'5 – dc19
DNLM/DLC
for Library of Congress 89-1327
CIP

ISSN 0935-1906

 Typesetting: A. Collignon, Berlin. – Printing and Binding: Elsnerdruck, Berlin. – Cover design: Rudolf Hübler. – Printed in Germany.

This monograph is dedicated
to Professor Dr. H. G. W. Frohmüller
on the occasion of his sixtieth anniversary.

Contents

Introduction

R. Ackermann

Treatment of urinary obstruction usually caused by benign prostatic hyperplasia (BPH) is still regarded by the public as the most common ailment confronting an urologist today. Although this is only true to some extent, transurethral resection of the prostate gland for BPH is still one of the most frequent operations in most urological units. Observations obtained from autopsy studies show that more than 70% of males aged 70 or over have histopathologically confirmed BPH. This substantiates the fact, that BPH is the most frequent neoplastic disease in man.

From this point of view it is understandable why so many scientists over the last century have made enormous efforts to discover the etiological factors which are responsible for the development of BPH. Two long-standing observations are of special importance. The fact that BPH develops with increasing age and that it occurs only in the presence of functioning testes implies that aging and endocrinological factors are involved in the pathogenesis of BPH. Inspite of earlier detailed macroscopic and microscopic descriptions of the normal prostate and of the benign enlarged gland, only recently have these findings been related to functional characteristics. Several comparative studies have contributed considerably to a better understanding of the anatomy and functional organization of the gland. It is now well accepted that the more surgically oriented description of two lateral and one median lobe should no longer be used as an anatomical basis. The description of a periurethral supracollicular zone, a central zone and of a peripheral zone within the gland is based on biological characteristics. Here, in addition to a better understanding of the anatomy, the various tissue compartments of the gland are more precisely defined. Although the possible role of the stromal tissue in the pathogenesis of BPH was suggested by Reischauer as early as 1925, the importance of this tissue in the development of BPH has only recently been substantiated through the application of stereological methods. Apart from the epithelial and stromal tissue compartment, interest is increasingly focused on the extracellular matrix and its role in epithelial stromal interactions. In this context, the description and biochemical characterization of mitogenic factors which were first discovered in malignant prostatic tissue may be of considerable pathogenic relevance.

Although BPH does not develop in prepuberal castrated men, the role of androgens for the development of BPH is not clearly defined. A large number of publications on hormone levels, steroid receptors and steroid metabolism in BPH has yielded conflicting data which had not contributed to a better understanding of the disease.

For the urologist who is confronted with BPH in daily practice it is almost impossible to follow the wide spectrum of scientific approaches in defining the etiology of BPH. The fact is that operative intervention, mainly by transurethral resection, is the only effective mode of treatment for the patient suffering from BPH.

This requires the precise identification of those patients who may benefit from the operation. However, there are no simple and completely reliable tests available by which the result of the treatment can be predicted. Although the development of transurethral resection must be considered as one of the major achievements in urology in this century, the problem of treating these patients has certainly not yet been sufficiently resolved.

Progress in defining the pathogenic factors responsible for the development of BPH and the presence of risk factors involved in surgical therapy stimulated the search for an effective medical form of treatment. Inspite of an increasing number of clinical trials initiated in the recent past, an effective pharmacological therapy has not yet been discovered. In addition reliable objective criteria for the evaluation of treatment responses have yet to be defined.

It is obvious that an extensive exchange of information among scientists with interest in different biological aspects of the BPH, as well as among experimental investigators and clinicians is mandatory to solve some of the addressed problems.

It was the aim of this symposium to provide a forum in which both basic scientists and clinicians could exchange their thoughts and problems, each from his respective point of view. Even more it was the intention of experts in the field of BPH to honor Professor Hubert Frohmüller on the occasion of his 60th birthday for his contributions in the clinical management of BPH.

Transurethral prostatic surgery at the Mayo Clinic

D. C. Utz

It is a high honor for me to be present on this auspicious occasion to bring tribute to Herr Professor Hubert Frohmüller from my colleagues at the Mayo Clinic. Professor Frohmüller's accomplishments and contributions are well known to all of us. This is an opportunity for us to celebrate his exceptional attainments, reflect on the wise counsel and guidance he has given us and to emulate his unsurpassed devotion to our profession.

He joins, indeed, Plato's noble group of men who carried the light and handed it to others.

It was a sunny, early spring day in April 1907 in Rochester, Minnesota. Dr. William F. Braasch stepped out of his second-hand automobile, quite a rarity in those days, onto the unpaved, muddy street in front of the Masonic Temple Building. He was dusty and road-weary. It had taken him 2 days to travel the eighty miles from Minneapolis to this prairie village of 4500 people. He wondered what compelled him, a successful practitioner of internal medicine, to accept the invitation from a country surgeon, Dr. William J. Mayo, to visit this clinic or group practice of medicine composed of 11 practitioners. He had heard about this novel form of medical practice – a group or clinic or integrated association – and he was anxious to discuss with the Mayo Brothers its future possibilities as well as the unique opportunity to develop instrumental diagnosis.

During the interview, Doctor Mayo expressed the opinion that clinical information derived by our five senses is more accurate than the limited laboratory data available at that time. He said this was particularly true when instruments were used to visualize the interior spaces of the body. The information derived would be particularly helpful to a surgeon as he gathered diagnostic data, limited as roentgenographic studies were in those days, to avoid as much as possible unexpected discoveries after making an incision.

Dr. Will Mayo explained that all forms of endoscopy should be in the hands of a man who would in time become a knowledgeable and experienced specialist. He offered Doctor Braasch the position and it was accepted. The problem was, however, that the new man – Doctor Braasch – had not even seen an endoscope, much less a cystoscope. Fortunately he read German fluently and in this language almost all of the significant methodology of its day was described.

New Developments in Biosciences 5

Doctor Braasch [2] went about the novel responsibility of developing endoscopy at the young Mayo Clinic, but after a time realized the data he accumulated was deficient. He found that greater diagnostic accuracy and value could be achieved if the information was collated by a physician, who was familiar with the other clinical and laboratory information about the patient. He discussed this important viewpoint with Doctor Will, who was persuaded and proctoscopy and bronchial and esophageal endoscopy were established as free standing entities, the Department of Urology took birth.

The evolution of the "cold punch" for transurethral prostatic resection, like all urologic endoscopic instruments, was inaugurated by Bozzini, who in 1807 in Frankfurt, Germany, first conceived and performed examination of the bladder with an endoscope using light reflected from without down the barrel. Guthrie in 1834, lecturing in London, described the prostatic median bar and advocated incision by means of a catheter, which had a concealed knife.

Realizing the limitations of incision of tissue only, Mercier in 1836 designed an instrument incorporating a conical excisor, which removed small pieces of prostatic tissue at the posterior commissure. Prostatic resection had dawned.

In 1909, Young [8] commenting, "the amount of tissue removed at suprapubic operations is often so small that it seems ridiculous to have to perform a suprapubic operation for its removal," modified the Mercier instrument by creating a fenestrum on the convex surface in the direction of the beak. No visualization of tissue excised or hemostasis was possible; nevertheless, interest in the United States in transurethral surgery was aroused and the word "punch" was added to urologic nomenclature.

Because of lack of visualization of the surgical field and of any means of hemostasis, the practicality of this instrument was seriously limited. These limitations were, to some extent, surmounted by Braasch [1], who incorporated in his direct vision cystoscope (fig. 1) an inner tubular sheath, which provided adequate observation of the tissue as it was excised.

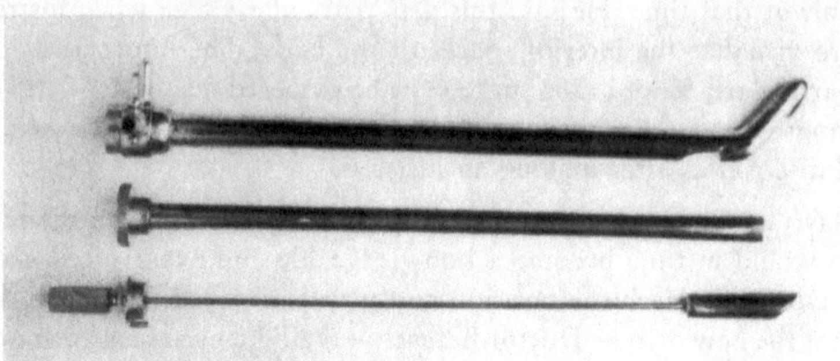

Fig. 1 Braasch's median bar excisor.

To solve the problem of electrocautery, Bumpus [3] modified the Braasch instrument to include an electrode on a guide so that it was no longer necessary to remove the cutting instrument and insert a cystoscope for hemostasis (fig. 2).

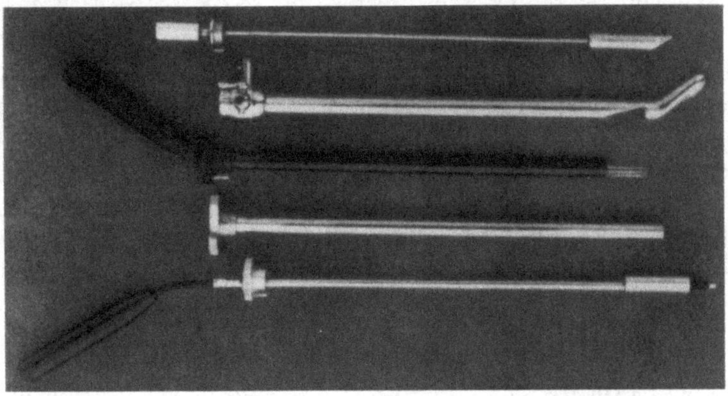

Fig. 2 Braasch cystoscope modified for prostatic resection.

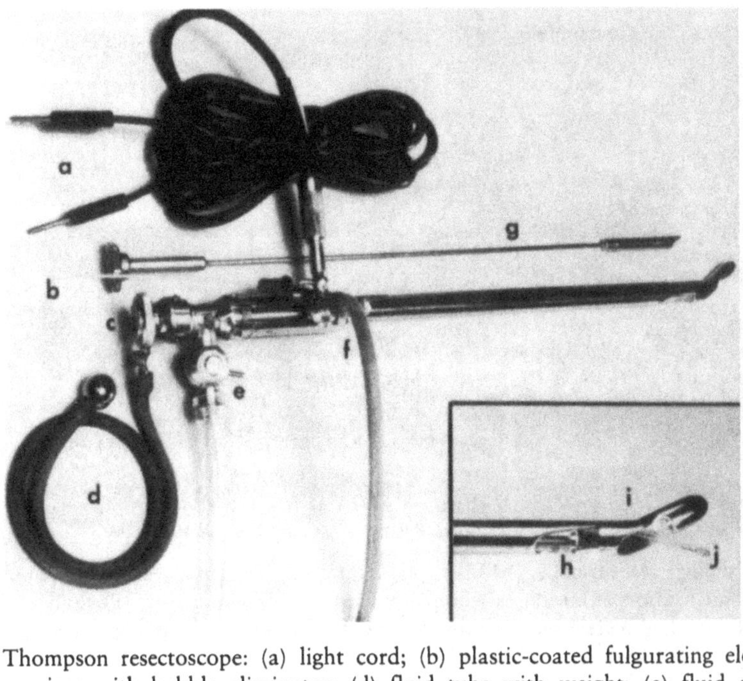

Fig. 3 Thompson resectoscope: (a) light cord; (b) plastic-coated fulgurating electrode; (c) eyepiece with bubble eliminator; (d) fluid tube with weight; (e) fluid outlet valve mounted on inner sheath; (g) obturator; (h) knife blade partially withdrawn; (i) fulgurating electrode.

In 1920, Dr. John Caulk of St. Louis developed the prototype of the hot loop resectoscope, but only after the experiments of Wappler Company with high frequency cutting current in 1922 was it possible for Davis and Stern and McCarthy to fabricate the electroresectoscope.

In 1935, Thompson [6] refined the direct vision resectoscope of Braasch and Bumpus to the extent that tissue to be removed could be inspected more precisely and excised under observation. With the Thompson instrument (fig. 3), a tubular knife on the end of a carrier, which also transports irrigating fluid, and moving within a 24 F, 27 F, or 30 F external sheath excises cores of tissue 1 – 2 grams in size. The irrigating fluid circulates through the eyepiece by exiting through a small aperture adjacent the glass and flowing down a rubber tube. Fulguration is carried out by means of an electrode assembled within the instrument. An outlet valve releases bladder content.

In 1973 Herr Professor Hubert Frohmüller [4] advanced the engineering of the Thompson by substituting fiber light illumination, adding the Lumina telescopic system, and altering the beak and the washer mechanism. The instrument is now well-known as the Frohmüller-Wolf resectoscope (fig. 4).

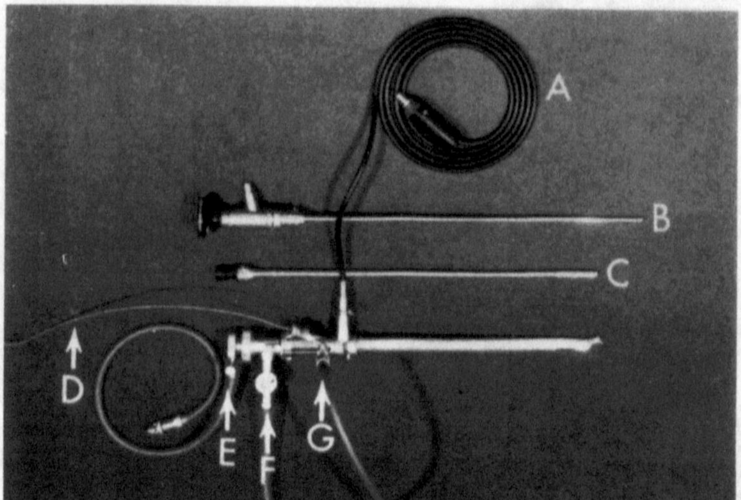

Fig. 4 Frohmüller resectoscope: (A) fiberoptic light cord; (B) lumina telescope; (C) obturator; (D) fulguration electrode; (E) eyepiece with bubble eliminator; (F) fluid outlet valve with attached plastic suction tube; (G) fluid inlet valve mounted on inner sheath.

Bladder evacuation apparatus

One of the exceptional advantages of the cold punch resectoscope is the capability of emptying the bladder of fluid and prostatic tissue rapidly and effectively by means of an attached suction system (fig. 5). A fluid outlet valve as large as the central caliber of the instrument accommodates the largest piece of tissue, about one gram, that can be resected. Components of this system are a firm plastic or rubber tube connected to the outlet valve of the resectoscope and a cylinder trap, which is stabilized inside a 5 gallon glass container. A vacuum is created and prostatic tissue is collected in the trap for frozen section analysis by the pathologists. The content of blood loss in the irrigating fluid can be calculated by the method of Litin & Emmett [5].

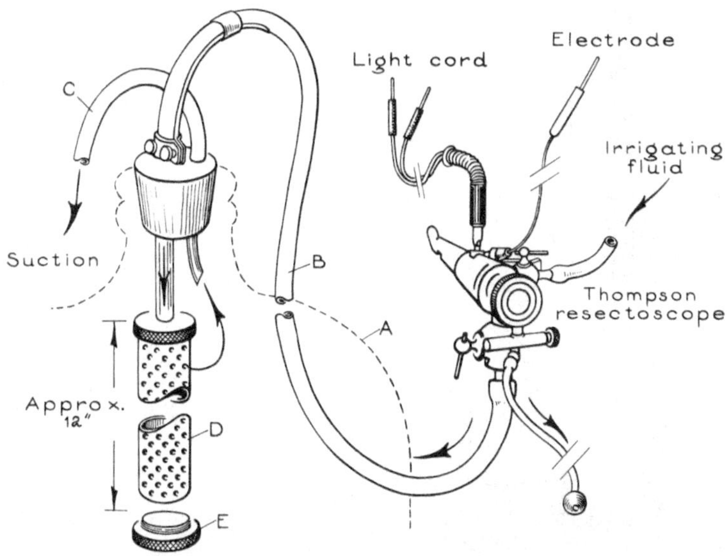

Fig. 5 Suction apparatus: (A) five-gallon collecting bottle (dotted line); (B) outlet tube that carries bloody irrigating fluid and cut pieces of tissue from bladder to collecting bottle; (C) suction tube connected to vacuum line; (D) trap that filters prostatic tissue from fluid. At conclusion of operation, trap is removed, lid (E) is unscrewed, and cut pieces of tissue are removed. (Litin, R. B., J. L. Emmett: Proc. Staff Mtg. Mayo Clin. *34* (1959) 158.)

Irrigating fluid

An essential component of the irrigating fluid system for the cold punch resectoscope is a relatively high, constant pressure to ensure adequate flow permitting clear vision through the instrument. The larger volume of nonhemolytic irrigating fluid that this instrument can accommodate affords an outstanding advantage of a clear field of vision even in the presence of sharp bleeding.

Preparatory procedure

Either prior or after cystoscopy, the Otis bougies, sizes 24 F to 30 F are passed initially to calibrate the urethra. If the 26 F Otis bougie does not pass, the urethra is dilated or an internal urethrotomy with the Otis urethrotome is carried out (fig. 6).

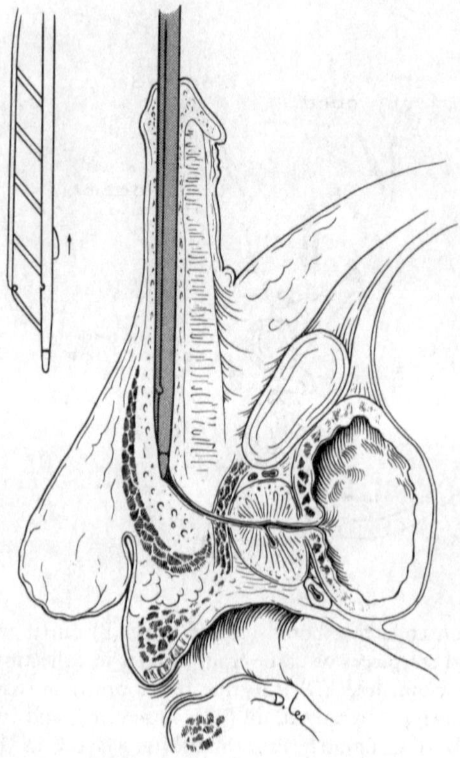

Fig. 6 Detail of Otis urethrotome and position in urethra.

Cystoscopy is performed. If the clinical impression of significant prostatic obstruction is confirmed, the urethra is prepared for passage of the resectoscope. An internal urethrotomy is performed if a 30 F Otis bougie encounters resistance in the urethra distal to the membranous segment.

There are three calibers of the punch resectoscope: 24 F, 28 F and 30 F. The 28 F instrument is most often used and the 30 F is generally reserved for adenomas larger than 100 grams. The smaller caliber is practical for younger patients with an obstructed vesical neck.

Technique of resection

The basic principles of transurethral resection are relatively the same, irrespective of whether the loop or punch resectoscope is employed. There are, however, some features of the cold punch procedure that should be understood.

Of special importance is the fact that prostatic tissue must be presented in the fenestrum of the resectoscope in order to be excised (fig. 7). To accomplish this, pressure is exerted by the left arm on the instrument. By using the urogenital diaphragm as a fulcrum, a lever action is obtained. In the final stages of the operation, resection of the median lobe tissue in a pocketed urethra is facilitated by digital rectal pressure against the posterior surface of the prostate.

There are four essential maneuvers involved in the cold punch technique. The first motion (fig. 8 a) is the identification of the segment of tissue to be resected.

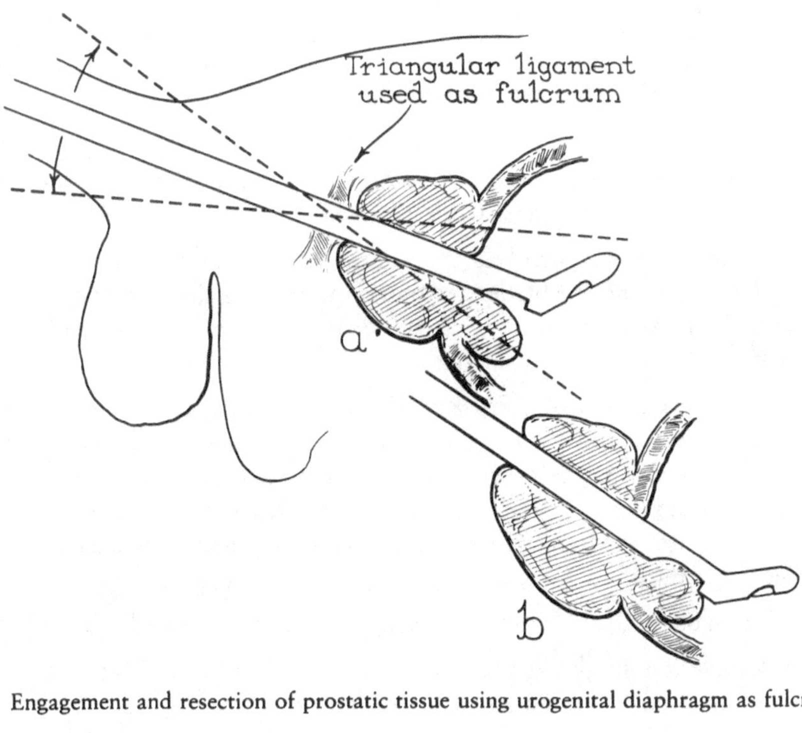

Fig. 7 Engagement and resection of prostatic tissue using urogenital diaphragm as fulcrum.

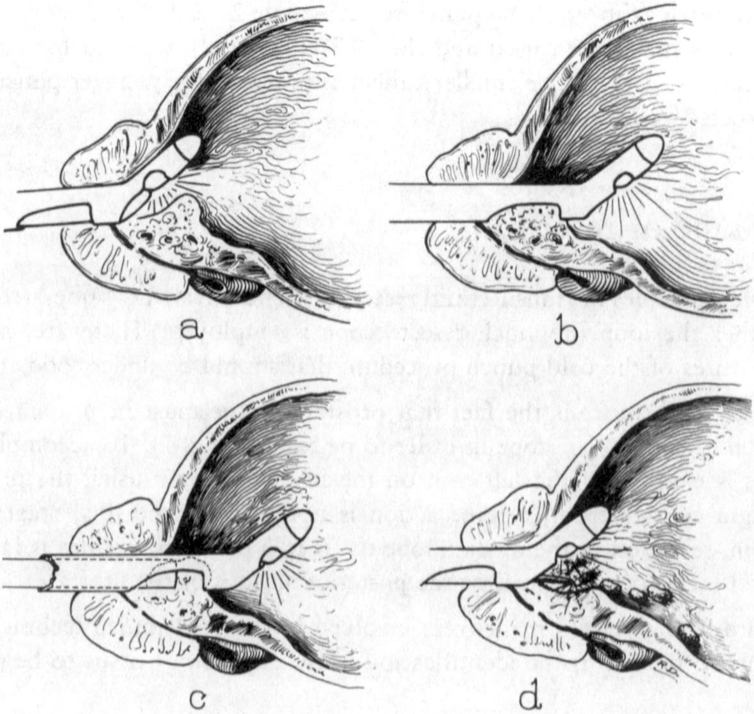

Fig. 8 Resection technique: (a) examination of prostatic tissue to be excised; (b) engagement of tissue in opened fenestra; (c) excision of tissue as knife is thrust forward to close fenestra; (d) electrofulguration of spurting vessels.

The inlet irrigating-fluid valve is opened fully, and the knife is in the home or closed position so that the fenestrum is closed.

The next step (fig. 8 b) involves the engagement of tissue. The instrument is advanced 2 – 3 cm and the blade is withdrawn, opening the fenestrum. The tissue is engaged by pressure on the resectoscope, and the prostatic tissue is secured in the fenestrum.

During the third maneuver (fig. 8 c), the inner sheath containing the tubular blades is thrust forward with a rapid, determined movement, excising the prostatic tissue. This portion of the prostate is propelled into the bladder by the stream of irrigating fluid through the opening near the beak of the instrument. When the bladder is distended, the tissue with the irrigating fluid is evacuated by closing the inlet irrigating-fluid valve and opening the outlet valve.

Finally, the most actively bleeding vessels are electrofulgurated (fig. 8 d).

At the completion of the operation, either a 22 F or 24 F irrigating retention catheter is inserted and maintained for 48 hours.

Discussion

Controversy over which type of instrument is superior – the hot loop or cold punch resectoscope – is simply pedantic and trivial.

Both instruments have their advantages and disadvantages, and excellent prostatic resections can be done by experienced urologists with either instrument. It is probably true, however, that few urologists are competent in the use of both instruments for prostatic resection.

To those trained in direct-vision cystoscopy, the use of the Frohmüller resectoscope is a natural. The unmagnified clear view of structures even in the presence of sharp bleeding, the tactile appreciation of tissue consistency, and the facility of removing resected tissue and irrigating fluid in the bladder seem to be distinct advantages.

Eighty years ago the young man who stepped out of his second-hand car on to the dusty street in Rochester, Minnesota, gave birth to the Department of Urology at the Mayo Clinic.

But with all of Doctor Braasch's keen sense of the significance of the changing times, he could not have envisioned in any way the influence of his contribution to urology.

A creative tradition developed within his Department by virtue of a succession of urologists gifted with consummate skill in urologic diagnosis and surgery.

Of these persons and others at the Mayo Clinic, Dr. W. J. Mayo was moved to remark: "These heroic men whose life work marked epochs in medicine we think of as individuals, but what they accomplished singly was perhaps of less importance than the inspiration they gave to the group of men who followed them."

The Clinic is especially proud of its contribution to the development of one of the most significant surgical procedures of the century, transurethral prostatic resection.

The road to acceptance was not easy. Doctor Thompson remarked in 1933 [7]: "I wish to assert that transurethral resection deserves the respect of everyone. It is an operation difficult to perform and can be done skillfully only by a good cystoscopist after gradual development of technique. Equipment must be complete, the operation must be as conservative as is consistent with a good result and postoperative observation should extend throughout the period of healing."

Year by year the popularity of the operation grew. In a 10 year period between 1932 – 1942, 8.800 transurethral resections were performed. But in a twenty-four year period, 1933 – 1957 almost 27.000 resections were done. About 1.000 operations a year are now done with a mortality rate of less than 0.1 percent.

The suprapubic prostatectomy of the 1920s, involving a mortality as high as 15 – 20% before the advent of antibacterial therapy and often involving a two-stage procedure, surrendered to transurethral resection with a mortality index even in those days of 2% with high risk patients over the age of 80.

The final argument with the skeptics, who deprecated the new operation as a primitive apple coring procedure, was conquered by Thompson, who showed that a transurethral prostatic resection removed just as much adenoma as the suprapubic operation often called a "prostatectomy."

As evidence of the superiority of prostatic transurethral resection, a team of physicians from the Mayo Clinic was selected to perform this operation on the President of the United States in January, 1987.

A successful operation was achieved and the patient was dismissed from the hospital on the third postoperative day. It was a tall occasion for me.

This day we are assembled to share our experiences, to impart our knowledge and to honor Herr Professor Hubert Frohmüller about whom Dr. Will Mayo's remarks in 1932 are especially pertinent: "What a man may do with his hands is small compared with what he can do to implant ideals and scientific spirit in many men, who in endless chains will carry on the same endeavor."

References

[1] Braasch, W. F.: Median bar excisor. JAMA *70* (1918) 758.
[2] Braasch, W. F., C. C. Thomas: Early Days in the Mayo Clinic. Springfield, IL. 1969.
[3] Bumpus, H. C., Jr.: Transurethral prostatic resection, Br. J. Urol. *4* (1932) 105.
[4] Frohmüller, H.: Direktsichtinstrumente in der Urologie. Verhandlungsbericht der Deutschen Gesellschaft für Urologie. Springer-Verlag, Berlin 1973.
[5] Litin, R. B., J. L. Emmett: Method of measuring blood loss during transurethral resection when nonhemolytic irrigating solutions are employed. Proc. Staff Mayo Clinic *34* (1959) 158.
[6] Thompson, G. J.: A new direct vision resectoscope. Urol. Cuta. Rev. *39* (1935) 545.
[7] Thompson, G. J.: Factors of safety in prostatic resection. J. Urol. *30* (1933) 525.
[8] Young, H. H.: A new procedure (punch operation) for small prostatic bars and contracture of the prostatic orifice. JAMA 9 (1913) 112.

Morphological aspects of the human prostate and the development of benign prostatic hyperplasia

G. Aumüller

Abstract

Different concepts of the normal anatomy and functional organization of the human prostate are presented and related to endocrine principles studied in experimental animals such as the dog and the rat. Contrary to the previous model of prostatic lobes, the current view of the inner structure of the gland is the discrimination of a periurethral supracollicular zone, a central zone surrounding the ejaculatory ducts and inserted in a wedgelike manner into the peripheral zone and made up of relatively simple-configurated acini. The functional interdependence and relationship between the stroma and the epithelium observed during embryological development, postnatal maturation and under certain pathological conditions has lead to the concept of the functional prostatic unit, which is useful for the explanation of prostatic growth and the expression of specific genes. Of particular importance with respect to glandular or stromal proliferation is the recent detection of different growth factors present in the prostate. In this review some peculiarities of prostatic smooth muscle are presented and are discussed with regard to current hypotheses on epithelial-stromal interactions in the control of gene expression in the prostate.

Internal organization of the human prostate

The traditional description of prostatic lobes (middle, lateral, anterior) was based on embryological considerations of Lowsley [20]. Several differing definitions of prostatic lobes have been developped subsequently [10, 40] which were not congruent.

In a series of papers McNeal [24, 25, 27] has criticized these older descriptions, and has developed a model based on certain dissection strategies and embryological observations. It envisages four subdivisions of the gland: 1. the non-glandular stroma, 2. the peripheral zone, 3. the central zone and 4. the preprostatic segment. A slightly modified view has been described by Altenähr et al. [1] and has been adopted to some recent findings in figure 1.

New Developments in Biosciences 5

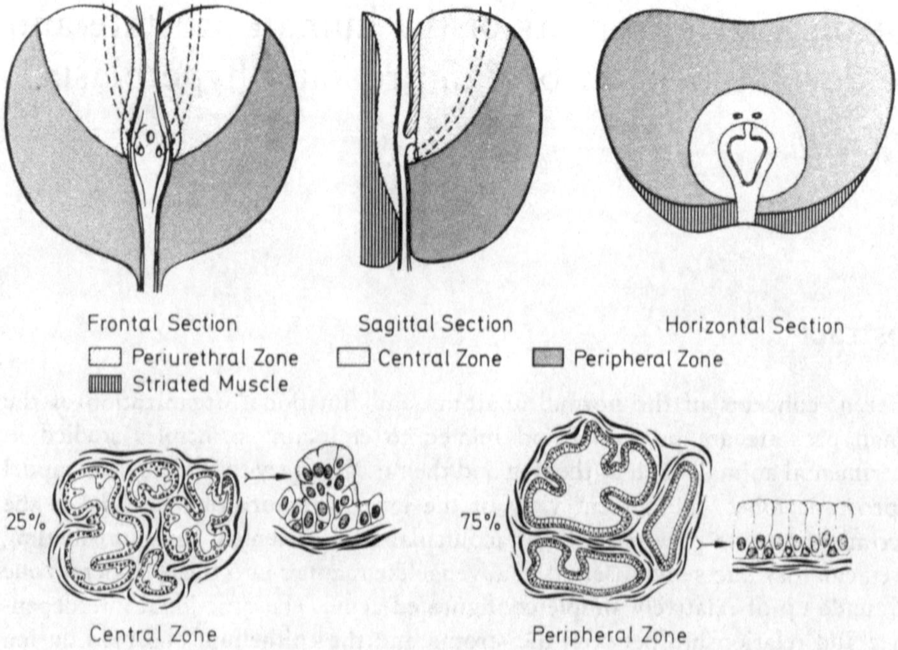

Fig. 1 Internal structure of the human prostate according to McNeal [24, 25] and Altenähr [1].

Most prostatic cancers are suggested to develop within the peripheral zone, i. e. that portion of the gland, the ducts of which radiate laterally from the urethra. They surround the central zone, a wedge-shaped group of ducts, arising close to the orifices of the ejaculatory ducts. The preprostatic region described by McNeal is the urethral segment proximal to the verumontanum which is kinked anteriorly to the distal segment. Duct development is aborted here, sometimes allowing the formation of an anterior "notch" [28], producing an only small transition zone and short periurethral ducts piercing into the periurethral sphincter. These ducts are suggested to form the primary site of development of benign prostatic hyperplasia (BPH).

There is growing evidence of a functional heterogeneity within the prostatic secretory duct system. In the canine prostate, for instance, considerable fine structural differences exist between the periurethral prostatic ducts and the peripheral glands [3] and similar observations have been made in the human prostate. The numer of epithelial cells containing the estrogen receptor [35], is much higher in the periurethral ducts, where close to the urethra endocrine cells are observed [7, 9, 34]. Another line of evidence for functional heterogeneity within the prostatic ducts comes from embryological observations. Sugimura et al. [38] showed that levels of DNA synthetic activity vary considerably within the (mouse) prostate on a regional basis. This finding is consistent with our own observations of a relatively long persistence of undifferentiated non-secretory acini during puberty at the peripheral tips of the gland ducts close to the dorsal capsule [5].

The prostatic functional unit

Morphological, functional and embryological studies have pointed to the highly differentiated interaction between various structures of prostatic stroma and prostatic epithelium. Both compartments therefore have been taken together, forming the so-called Prostatic Functional Unit (fig. 2). It encompasses the secretory cells and their adjacent auxiliary structures, such as the basal cells, the basal lamina, the capillaries, fibrocytes, smooth muscle cells, free connective tissue cells, nerve axons and lymphatics which are all destined to provide the secretory cells with the required oxygen, hormones, energy, ions, transmitter signals and to remove metabolites from the cells. While previously the basal cells have been claimed to represent non-differentiated stem-cells, this suggestion now is mostly abandoned [2]. Instead, our recent observation that smooth muscle-specific actin together with cytokeratin is present in the basal cells is much in favour of a myoepithelial function of these cells as previously suggested by Rowlatt and Franks [33]. Secretory cells in the human prostate form from non-secretory columnar cells during puberty. Maturation of prostatic secretory function is readily determined by the immunohistochemical visualization on one major secretory protein, such as acid phosphatase. In the prepubertal gland only a few cells of the large ducts are immunoreactive. The older the individual, the more intense becomes the reaction of the peripheral parts of the gland ducts, accompanied by a more elaborate formation of the glandular structure. The latter acquires its definite shape at the age of about 20 years. In elderly men, the structural complexity is mostly lost and there is a considerable variation in the intensity of secretory immunoreactivity.

Some authors have claimed a regulatory role of prostatic secretion on cellular proliferation, but only the recent finding of prostatic growth factors has substantiated this idea [14, 17, 21, 37]. A homeostatic constraint mechanism of prostatic growth has been claimed by Bruchovsky et al. [11].

An additional aspect has been brought into the discussion by Marriotti and Mawhinney [23]. They presume that in the fully developed (rat) prostate androgen stimulates the fibroblasts to production of collagen which provides the scaffold for growing epithelial cells. The increase of collagen were counteracted by a breakdown of collagen through the action of a collagenolytic enzyme secreted from the glandular cells.

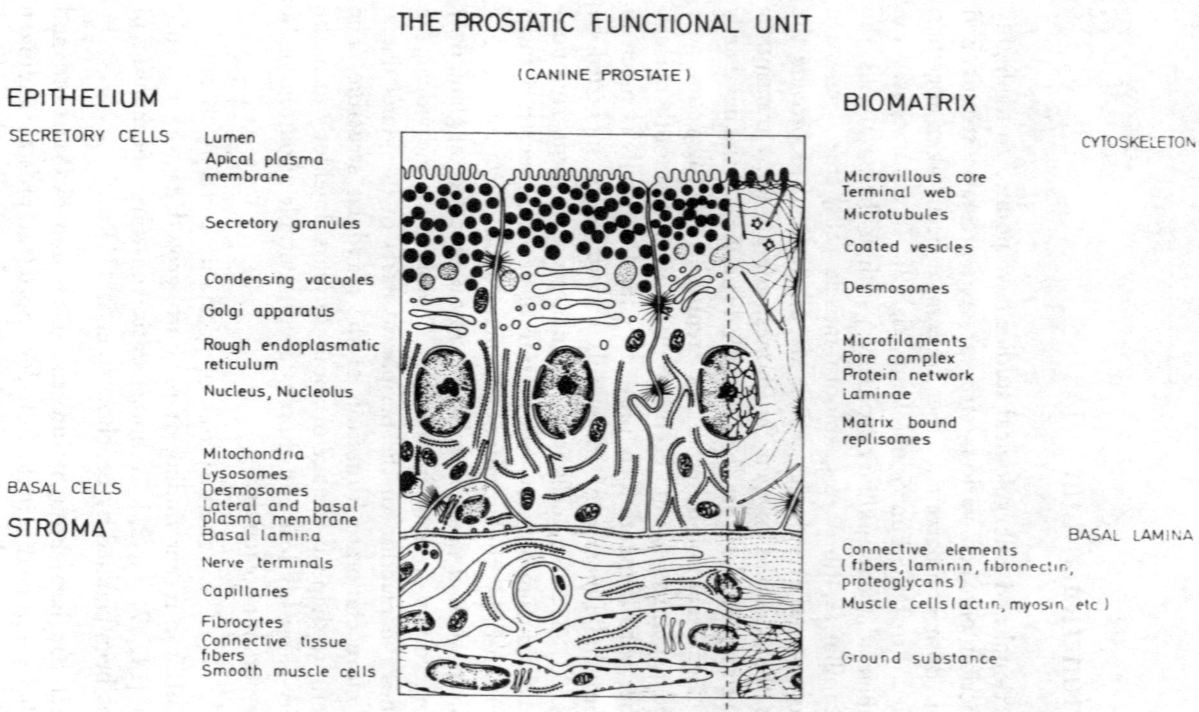

Fig. 2 The essential structural components forming the prostatic functional unit (from 2). The intracellular cytoskeleton and the extracellular matrix are shown at the right hand side forming a common superstructure.

A slightly different suggestion including some endocrine aspects, has been proposed by the present author [2]. Its basic idea is that the assumption of a bloodborne, freely diffusible chalone transmitted by prostatic cells is not necessary, but instead the regulation of cellular proliferation may be represented by secretory products of the respective cells. The products of normal functional activity of the gland would be a mitosis-inhibiting agent, effective when present above a certain threshold concentration. Quantitative intracellular reduction of this presumptive substance below its effective concentration during, e. g. autophagic processes or stimulated extrusion subsequent to androgenic or estrogenic challenge, would give a signal to the cell to divide, provided sufficient testosterone was availabe.

Stroma of the prostate

The great functional significance of prostatic stroma has been disclosed only in recent years. The most obvious structure of prostatic stroma are smooth muscle cells forming tiny sheaths around the acini, or, alternatively, broad strands, separating larger parts of the gland. In the organ of the adult, in stroma forms both a mechanically stabilizing factor, particularly in the preurethral and capsular parts of the gland, as well as a motorial element in the expulsion of secretion. The identification of the stroma as the dominant component during development has led to detailed studies of prostatic stroma separated from the epithelium [12, 18, 19, 30]. Considerable differences between both components have been detected, such as the differential distribution of steroid receptors, steroid metabolites and enzymes. Recent observations of smooth muscle-derived growth factors throw new light on prostatic smooth muscle as one major component in the development of benign prostatic hyperplasia. The ultrastructure of prostatic smooth muscle cells is rather identical in various species and location within the gland. The cytoplasm of these cells is occupied chiefly by fine filaments (6 nm in diameter) that are mainly oriented parallel to the long axis of the cell. Spindle shaped dense bodies are scattered throughout the course of the filaments. The latter extend into dense plaques subjacent to the plasma membrane. The arrangement and distribution of cell organelles is nearly identical with that in seminal vesicle smooth muscle cells. Surface vesicles (caveolae) have been found arranged in clusters separated from each other by smooth areas of the cell surface seen on freeze-etch replicas. Each cell is surrounded by a basal lamina of about 50 nm in thickness. Cell contacts are infrequent in peripheral prostatic stroma. Intermediate junctions are rather frequent between smooth muscle cells close to or within the muscle layer of the prostatic urethra. Here, cells are often intermingled with a dense feltwork of elastic fibers. Prostatic smooth muscle is innervated by preferentially adrenergic nerves [9, 29] which in addition contain enkephalins [41]. The presence of alpha-adrenoceptors has been demonstrated [16] in pharmacological experiments using isolated strips of prostatic tissue.

Hormone-dependence of prostatic smooth muscle

Rohr et al. [31, 32] and Bartsch et al. [8] have shown in a series of papers that in the absence of androgens, estrogens are capable to transform prostatic smooth muscle cells into "activated" cells. The concept of "activated" smooth muscle has been developed from earlier observations of Chamley-Campbell et al. [13] in vascular smooth muscle cells, where at least two different phenotypic states of smooth muscle dependent on age are observed. In the developing organism the cells have a fibroblast-like appearance, divide, and secrete extracellular matrix components; at this stage they are referred to as being in "synthetic" phenotype. In the adult the smooth muscle cells become highly differentiated and specialized, contracting in response to chemical and mechanical stimuli; at this stage they are referred to as being in a "contractile" state. An ultrastructural study devoted to phenotypic alterations of canine prostatic smooth muscle after a six-months treatment with androgens and estrogens and/or antiandrogens and antiestrogens has been performed in castrated dogs [4]. Compared to the normal conditions in the prostate of castrated dogs the size of the individual smooth muscle cell is clearly reduced, along with a decrease in microfilaments and dense bodies. The cells are situated close to each other forming thick bands interspersed between strands of connective tissue. Androgen substitution with 3 α-androstenediol, even in the presence of estrogen and antiestrogen, is capable of reversing the atrophic changes. In the case of diminished androgen-levels and increased estrogen levels, signs of metabolic and structural alteration develop, initially in form of clusters of glycogen surrounding the perinuclear zone. In castrated animals treated simultaneously with androstenediol, the antiandrogen cyproterone acetate and estradiol, an enormous accumulation of lipid occurred in the perinuclear zone of the smooth muscle cells, replacing a large proportion of cytoplasmic organelles and myofilaments (fig. 3). Similar alterations occurred in adjacent fibroblasts. Estrogen was identified as the compound inducing structural and functional dedifferentiation of prostatic smooth muscle cells in castrated animals treated exclusively with estradiol. Most cells showed fatty degeneration and only few cells remained in contractile state. Estrogen-mediated dedifferentiation of prostatic smooth muscle cells is also observed in castrated dogs treated with an androgen that is practially metabolized to estrogen by the enzyme aromatase [6]. In initial stages of androstenedione treatment, alterations in smooth muscle cells are observed resembling those of the synthetic state of vascular smooth muscle.

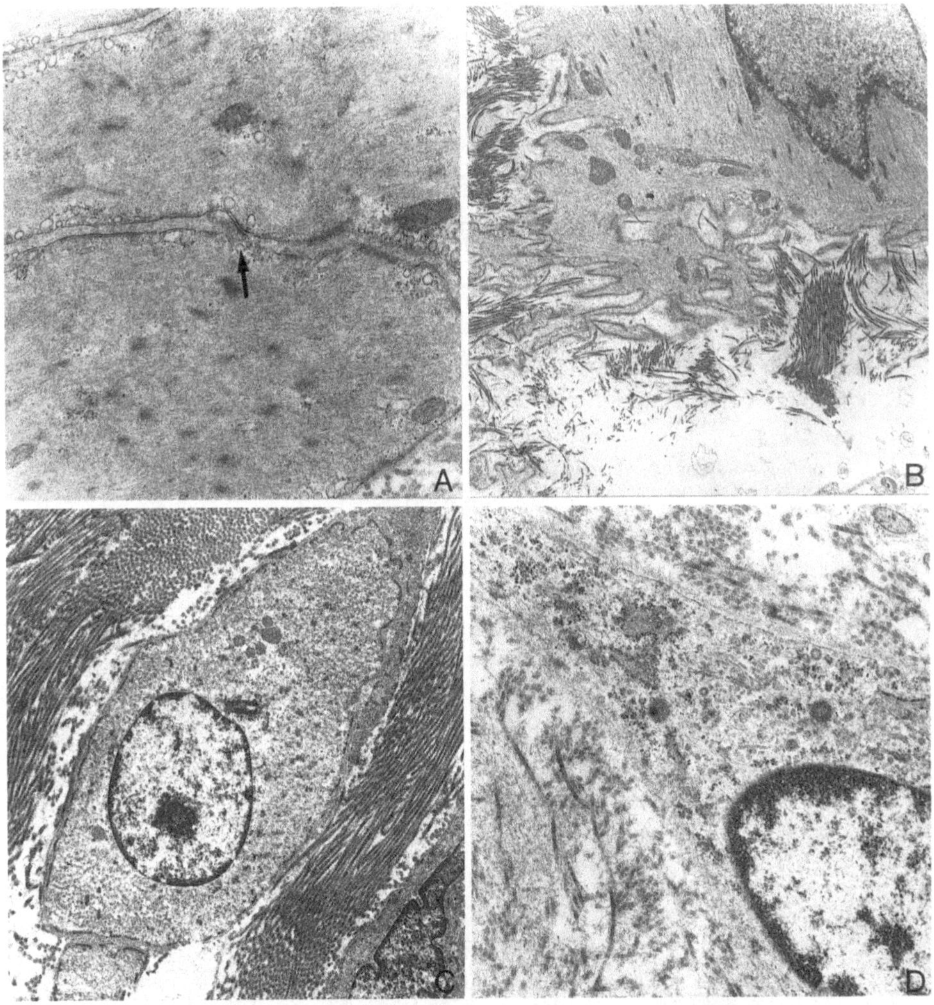

Fig. 3 Hormone-dependence of the ultrastructural organization of prostatic smooth muscle: A. The normal fine structure shown in smooth muscle of the rat lateral prostate. Arrow: intermediate junction. B. 14 days after castration, the cells are shrunken. C. Prostatic smooth muscle cell from a castrated dog treated with androstanediol, estradiol and tamoxifen. The cell is slightly activated. D. Canine prostatic cell from a castrated, estradiol-treated animal. The cell has switched from the contractile to the metabolic state.

It is tempting to speculate that a changed endocrine situation in the aged human leads to an increased number in "activated" or "synthetic" smooth muscle cells, effecting certain epithelial-stromal interactions usually operating during the onset of prostatic development and resulting in benign prostatic hyperplasia [15, 26].

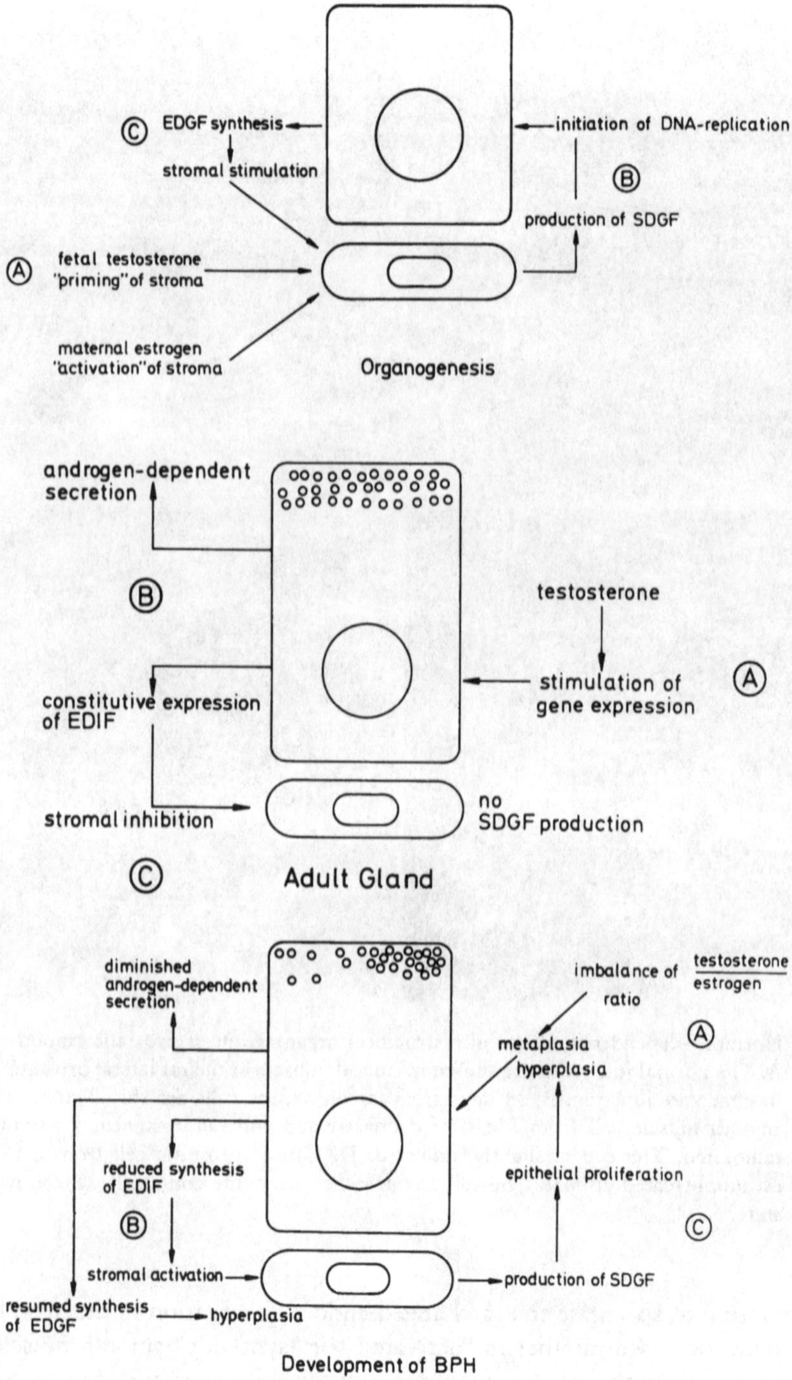

Fig. 4 A modified sketch of the Tenniswood-hypothesis [39]. See text for details.

Hypotheses on epithelial-stromal interacting during BPH development

The recent findings of an interdependence between synthesis of platelet derived growth factor, heparin-like glycosaminoglycans and vascular smooth muscle growth [22, 36] should encourage upcoming scientific efforts to find experimental support for a hypothesis on the role of epithelial-stromal interactions in the control of prostatic gene expression, recently advanced by Tenniswood [39] and illustrated in slightly modified sketches (fig. 4). This hypothesis proposes the existence of three factors, two growth factors, namely a "stromally derived growth factor" (SDGF) and an "epithelially derived growth factor" (EDGF), and one inhibiting factor, "epithelially derived inhibiting factor" (EDIF) which together modulate gene expression in the prostate during development and adult function. The hypothesis also attempts to explain the etiology of certain prostatic diseases: if, for example the production of SDGF and EDGF is not coordinately regulated, the overproduction of one or the other would be expected to lead to hyperplastic structures that are either predominantly epithelial (if SDGF is in excess) or stromal (if EDGF is in excess). In the normal adult gland the constitutive expression of EDIF by the epithelial cells would repress SDGF gene expression in the stromal cells. This would prevent replication in both cell types enabling them to express continually the genes for steroid metabolism and secretion. In this hypothesis stroma cells, especially smooth muscle cells, have been taken into account as a morphologically and functionally stable and differentiated cellular entity. As has been shown above, however, this is not the case (as likewise is not the case for the epithelium), but instead there are considerable phenotypic alterations of the smooth muscle cells depending on the hormonal situation and reflecting altered functional activities of the cells.

Future studies must address the question, whether an estrogen-induced shift of smooth muscle cells from a "contractile" to a "synthetic" state would initiate the production of a stromally derived growth factor or any other imbalance in the system effecting proliferation either of smooth muscle cells or glandular structures during the development of benign prostatic hyperplasia.

References

[1] Altenähr, E.: Pathologie des Prostatakarzinoms. In: H. Klosterhalfen, E. Altenähr, H. D. Franke (eds): Das Prostatakarzinom. Pathologie – Diagnostik – Therapie, pp. 1–72. Thieme, Stuttgart – New York 1982.

[2] Aumüller, G.: Morphologic and endocrine aspects of prostatic function. The Prostate *4* (1983) 195–214.

[3] Aumüller, G., E. Stofft, U. Tunn: Fine structure of the canine prostatic complex. Anat. Embryol. *160* (1980) 327–340.

[4] Aumüller, G., P. J. Funke, A. Hahn et al.: Phenotypic modulation of the canine prostate after long-term treatment with androgens and estrogens. The Prostate *3* (1982) 361–373.

[5] Aumüller, G., J. Seitz, W. Bischof: Immunohistochemical study on the initiation of acid phosphatase secretion in the human prostate. J. Androl. *4* (1983) 183–191.

[6] Aumüller, G., U. F. Habenicht, M. F. El Etreby: Pharmacologically induced ultrastructural and immunohistochemical changes in the prostate of castrated dogs. The Prostate *11* (1987) 211–218.

[7] Azzopardi, J.-G., D. J. Evans: Argentaffin cells in prostatic carcinoma: differentiation from lipofuscin and melanin in prostatic epithelium. J. Pathol. *104* (1971) 247–251.

[8] Bartsch, G., A. Bruengger, D. P. DeKlerk et al.: Light-microscopic stereologic analysis of spontaneous and steroid-induced canine prostatic hyperplasia. J. Urol. *137* (1987) 552–558.

[9] Baumgarten, H. G., B. Falck, A.-F. Holstein et al.: Adrenergic innervation of the human testis, epididymis, ductus deferens and prostate. Z. Zellforsch. *90* (1968) 81–95.

[10] Blacklock, N. J.: The morphology of the parenchyma of the prostate. Urol. Res. *5* (1977) 155–158.

[11] Bruchovsky, N., B. Lesser, P. Rennie: Control of the concentration and distribution of dihydrotestosterone in prostatic cells. In: M. Goland (ed.): Normal and abnormal growth of the prostate, pp. 125–143. Charles C. Thomas, Springfield, JL., 1975.

[12] Bruchovsky, N., M. G. McLoughlin, R. S. Rennie et al.: Partial characterisation of stromal and epithelial forms of 5 α-reductase in human prostate. In: G. P. Murphy, A. A. Sandberg, J. P. Karr (eds): The Prostatic Cell: Structure and Function, Part A, pp. 161–175. Liss Inc., New York 1981.

[13] Chamley-Campbell, J., G. R. Campbell, R. Ross: Phenotype-dependent response of cultured aortic smooth muscle to serum mitogens. J. Cell Biol. *89* (1981) 379–383.

[14] Crabb, J. W., L. G. Armes, S. A. Carr et al.: Complete primary structure of prostatotropin, a prostate epithelial cell growth factor. Biochemistry *25* (1986) 4988–4993.

[15] Cunha, G. R., L. W. K. Chung, J. M. Shannon et al.: Stromal-epithelial interactions in sex differentiation. Biol. Reprod. *22* (1980) 19–42.

[16] Hieble, J. P., A. J. Boyce, M. Caine: Comparison of the α-adrenoceptor characteristics in human and canine prostate. Fed. Proc. *45* (1986) 2609–2614.

[17] Hierowski, M. T., W. M. McDonald, L. Dunn et al.: The partial dependency of human prostatic growth factor on steroid hormones in stimulating thymidine incorporation into DNA. J. Urol. *138* (1987) 909–912.

[18] Jung-Testas, I., M. T. Groyer, J. Bruner-Lorand et al.: Androgen and estrogen receptors in rat ventral prostate epithelium and stroma. Endocrinol. *109* (1981) 1287–1289.

[19] Krieg, M., G. Klötzl, J. Kaufmann et al.: Stroma of human benign prostatic hyperplasia: preferential tissue for androgen metabolism and estrogen binding. Acta Endocrinol. (Copenhagen) *96* (1981) 422–432.

[20] Lowsley, D. S.: The development of the human prostate gland with reference to the development of other structures at the neck of the urinary bladder. Am. J. Anat. *13* (1912) 299–349.

[21] Maehama, S., D. Li, H. Nanri et al.: Purification and partial characterization of prostate-derived growth factor. Proc. Natl. Acad. Sci. USA *83* (1986) 8162–8166.

[22] Majack, R. A., S. C. Cook, P. Bornstein: Platelet-derived growth factor and heparin-like glycosaminoglycans regulate thrombospondin synthesis and deposition in the matrix by smooth muscle cells. J. Cell Biol. *101* (1985) 1059–1070.

[23] Marriotti, A., M. Mawhinney: Preliminary studies of the hormonal control of male accessory sex organ epithelial collagen. In: G. P. Murphy, A. A. Sandberg, J. P. Karr (eds): The Prostatic Cell. Structure and Function, pp. 133 – 136. Liss Inc., New York 1981.
[24] McNeal, J. E.: Regional morphology and pathology of the prostate. Am. J. Clin. Pathol. *49* (1968) 347 – 357.
[25] McNeal, J. E.: The prostate and prostatic urethra: A morphologic synthesis. J. Urol. *107* (1972) 1008 – 1016.
[26] McNeal, J. E.: Origin and evolution of benign prostatic enlargement. Invest. Urol. *15* (1978) 340 – 345.
[27] McNeal, J. E.: Anatomy of the prostate: An historical survey of divergent views. The Prostate *1* (1980) 3 – 13.
[28] Myers, R. P., J.-R. Goellner, D. R. Cahill: Prostate shape, external striated urethral sphincter and radical prostatectomy: the apical dissection. J. Urol. *138* (1987) 543 – 550.
[29] Owman, Ch., N.-O. Sjöstrand: Short adrenergic neurons and catecholamine-containing cells in vas deferens and accessory male genital glands of different mammals. Z. Zellforsch. *66* (1965) 300 – 320.
[30] Robel, P., B. Eychenne, J.-P. Blondeau et al.: Characteristics of separated epithelial and stroma subfractions of prostate: II. Human Prostate. The Prostate *5* (1984) 255 – 268.
[31] Rohr, H. P., M. Oberholzer, G. Bartsch et al.: Morphometry in experimental pathology: Methods, baseline data, and applications. Int. Rev. exp. Path. *15* (1976) 233 – 325.
[32] Rohr, H. P., G. Bartsch, N. DeKlerk et al.: Light microscopic stereological analysis of experimental induction of dog prostatic hyperplasia. Arch. Androl. *2* (1979) Suppl. 1 (abstr.).
[33] Rowlatt, C., L. M. Franks: Myoepithelium in mouse prostate. Nature *202* (1964) 707 – 708.
[34] Sant'Agnese, P. A. di, K. L. de Mesy Jensen: Endocrine-paracrine cells of the prostate and prostatic urethra: an ultrastructural study. Hum. Pathol. *15* (1984) 1034 – 1041.
[35] Schulze, H., E. R. Barrack: Immunocytochemical localization of estrogen receptors in spontaneous and experimentally induced canine benign prostatic hyperplasia. The Prostate *11* (1987) 145 – 162.
[36] Sjölund, M., U. Hedin, Th. Sejersen et al.: Arterial smooth muscle cells express platelet-derived growth factor (PDGF) A chain mRNA, secrete a PDGF-like mitogen and bind exogenous PDGF in a phenotype- and growth state-dependent manner. J. Cell Biol. *106* (1988) 403 – 413.
[37] Story, M. T., F. Esch, S. Shimasaki et al.: Amino-terminal sequence of a large form of basic fibroblast growth factor isolated from human benign prostatic hyperplastic tissue. Biochem. Biophys. Res. Comm. *142* (1987) 702 – 709.
[38] Sugimura, Y., G. R. Cunha, A. A. Donjacour: Morphological and histological study of castration-induced degeneration and androgen-induced regeneration in the mouse prostate. Biol. Reprod. *34* (1986) 973 – 983.
[39] Tenniswood, M.: Role of epithelial-stromal interactions in the control of gene expression in the prostate: An hypothesis. The Prostate *9* (1986) 375 – 385.
[40] Tisell, L.-E., H. Salander: The lobes of the human prostate. Scand. J. Urol. Nephrol. *9* (1975) 185 – 191.
[41] Valaasti, A., J. Linnoila, A. Hervonen: Immunohistochemical demonstration of VIP [Met^5]- and [Leu^5]-enkephalin immunoreactive nerve fibres in the human prostate and seminal vesicles. Histochemistry *88* (1980) 89 – 98.

Stem cell organization of the prostate and the development of benign prostatic hyperplasia

J. T. Isaacs

Introduction

While benign prostatic hyperplasia (BPH) is the most common neoplastic disease in both man and dog, the exact etiology of this disorder in either species is presently unknown. Over the last 40 years, numerous theories have been postulated to explain the spontaneous development of BPH. Only two facts however have been well established for the disease in both species. The first is that the presence of functioning testes is required for the natural development [3, 16, 27, 32]. Whether the testes play a permissive or active role in the development of BPH is uncertain, however, the fact that pre-pubertal castration prevents the subsequent development of BPH suggests that there are at least some endocrinological determinants in the etiology of BPH. The second fact is that the incidence of BPH increases with advancing age such that nearly all men or dogs eventually develop BPH if they live long enough [5, 7, 27]. These two facts suggest that aging and endocrinological factors are indeed important in the process of BPH development, however, the exact manner in which these two factors are involved in the etiology of BPH is not clear.

In addition, studies have demonstrated that once BPH has developed, androgen ablation leads to a decrease in BPH size [4, 16, 17, 28]. Following androgen ablation, however, if a physiological androgen level is restored, the regressed BPH rapidly regrows to its abnormal size [4, 28]. This demonstrates that factor(s) within the hyperplastic gland itself, not merely systemic factors, are involved in BPH development and maintenance. In an attempt to identify the factor(s) involved in regulating prostate size, whether normal or hyperplastically enlarged, comparative studies on the organization of the prostate have been undertaken using the rat, dog, and human prostate.

The choice of these particular animal species is for the following reasons. In the dog, beside the spontaneous development of benign hyperplastic overgrowth of the prostate which occurs with increasing incidence with advancing age [7], BPH can be induced experimentally by means of exogeneous treatment of young dogs with androgen [12, 31]. Unlike the dog, the rat does not spontaneously develop

New Developments in Biosciences 5

BPH, nor can BPH be experimentally induced in this species regardless of type or extent of androgen treatment [6]. Therefore by comparing age related changes in a variety of parameters in the rat versus the dog and human, the essential nature of these changes with regard to BPH development can be evaluated.

Normal prostate as a steady-state self renewing system

An increase in cell number over time occurs whenever there is an imbalance between the rate of cell proliferation and cell death within any tissue, whether normal or neoplastic. This imbalance can be induced by either an increase in the cell proliferation and/or decrease in cell death. The prostate of the rat, dog, and man normally undergoes two distinct phases during the lifetime of the host. The first, or growth phase, begins at birth and continues until the prostate reaches its normal adult size [20]. If the host is castrated at birth, the proliferative growth of the prostate is completely blocked. These results clearly demonstrate that a physiological level of androgen is chronically required for the normal growth phase of the prostate.

The prostate normally continues to grow until it reaches its maximum adult size. When this size is reached, the gland normally ceases continuous net growth and a second maintenance phase of the prostate begins. During this maintenance phase the cells of the normal prostate are continuously turning over with time, with the rate of prostatic cell proliferation during this maintenance phase balanced by an equal rate of prostatic cell death such that neither involution nor overgrowth of the gland normally occurs with time. The normal adult prostate, during its maintenance phase, is thus an example of a steady-state self renewing tissue [21]. If an adult male whose prostate is in this steady-state maintenance condition is castrated, the serum testosterone levels rapidly decrease. As a result, the prostate rapidly involutes. This involution demonstrates that a physiological level of androgen is chronically required during the maintenance, as well as the earlier growth phase, of the normal prostate.

This continuous requirement for androgen is due to the fact that androgen chronically stimulates the rate of cell proliferation while simultaneously inhibiting the rate of cell death [19]. While the agonistic ability of androgen on prostatic cell proliferation has been well established by a variety of studies, the additional ability of androgen to agonistically inhibit the rate of cell death has only recently been fully appreciated [19]. Indeed, the rapid involution of prostate following castration is predominantly due to a major decreased antagonistic effect of androgen on prostatic cell death rather than to a major decreased agonistic effect of androgen on prostatic cell proliferation [19]. After a period following castration, the rate of prostatic cell loss eventually slows dramatically and is no longer exponential. Indeed, a percentage of the prostatic cells initially present before castration are able to survive long term castration. This demonstrates that the prostate is not homogeneous, but is instead, heterogeneously composed of both androgen-dependent cells (i. e. cells which are eliminated following castration) and androgen-independent cells (i. e. cells which survive following castration).

In an intact adult male, the supply of androgen regulates a balance between prostatic cell death and proliferation such that neither continuing involution nor overgrowth of the gland normally occurs. This is clearly illustrated by the fact that it is possible to titrate and maintain prostatic cell number from its lowest value in untreated castrated hosts to graded levels depending upon the serum testosterone level maintained in the treated hosts [25]. For example, for the rat, there is a highly significant linear positive correlation between the prostatic DHT content which is produced at various serum testosterone concentrations and the eventual steady-state content of total prostatic cells [25].

These results demonstrate that the prostatic cell content is, in general, proportional to the prostatic content of DHT, at least between the range of DHT levels observed in castrated hosts up to the levels observed for intact control males. In castrated male rats, the serum testosterone level can be raised to greater than twice the normal level of untreated intact animals which results in an abnormal elevation (2-fold) in the prostatic DHT content. Such treatment, while increasing the prostatic DHT content twofold above normal, however, can not induce any further increase in prostatic cell number above that seen in the untreated intact control rats, even if such treatments were continued for several months [6, 25]. These results demonstrated that total prostatic cell content is dependent upon a critical level of androgenic stimulation; however, excessive androgenic stimulation alone cannot induce the prostatic cell number to abnormally increase continuously in the rat [6, 25]. Therefore, what actually controls the upper limit of prostatic cell content in the rat.

Stem cell model for the organization of the prostate

In many other steady-state self-renewing tissue systems (i. e. skin, bone marrow, testes, gut, etc.), control over the total cell content of a tissue is determined by the number of self-renewing stem cells contained within the tissue itself. A stem cell is defined as a cell type capable of extensive self-renewal (i. e. proliferative) in spite of physiological or accidental removal or loss of cells from the population. The fraction of the proliferative pool of cells in the renewing prostate that are stem cells is unknown. It had been assumed that the stem cell fraction is close to 1 on the basis of thymidine labeling of the epithelial cells of the involuted prostate of long-term castrated animals in response to exogenous androgenic stimulation [26]. Androgen cycling experiments, however, suggest that the fraction of prostatic cells which are stem cells is low, with the majority of the cell production within the gland being due instead to the proliferation of sub-classes of cells which have only a limited self-renewal capacity [21]. This conclusion is based upon the fact, that by using a method of cyclically inducing prostate involution and then restoration of the gland it is possible to induce >60 population doubling in the rat ventral prostate. Even after more than 60 population doublings, however, the ventral prostate is completely able to repopulate itself normally [21].

These *in vivo* findings are in direct contrast to the findings obtained with *in vitro* cultured cells. It has been well documented that normal (i. e. nonneoplastic) cells, when they are cultured, have only a limited number of population doublings which they can undergo *in vitro* before they lose their proliferative potential [15]. In addition, there is a good correlation between maximum life span of various vertebrate species and the maximum number of population doublings which their fibroblasts can undergo *in vitro*. For rodent fibroblasts, this senescence occurs after less than 10 population doublings; for human fibroblasts it occurs after 50 ± population doublings [14]. How then can the rat prostate cells undergo more than 60 *in vivo* population doublings and still retain its normal vigorous ability to restore its total cell number following androgen withdrawal? These results are highly paradoxical if restoration of the involuted prostate is due solely to the continuous proliferation of only a single class of cells (i. e. stem cells) in the gland. Alternatively, these results suggest that additional subclasses of amplifying cells capable of limited proliferation must also be present along with stem cells in the involuted prostate. While these amplifying cells originate from stem cells and can proliferate for only limited numbers of cell division, these proliferations result in a major amplification in the total number of cells present. This amplification can be extensive, for example, if the amplifying cells can divide five times, this produces a 32-fold amplification in total cell number; if they can divide 10 times, this produces a 1.000-fold amplification. Such amplification results in the stem cells being a minority population in the tissue. Thus restoration of the involuted prostate after castration by exogenous androgen probably involves only a small, if any, increase in the rate of stem cell renewal, the major restoration in cell number being due to the increase proliferation of the pool of preexisting amplifying cells. Such a model for prostatic cell renewal is presented in Figure 1. In this model attention is drawn to the fact that the amplifying cells are androgen-independent since they are able to exist even in long-term castrated animals. This point is emphasized by the fact that it is possible to castrate male adults and allow an extended period (i. e. > years) before replacing androgen

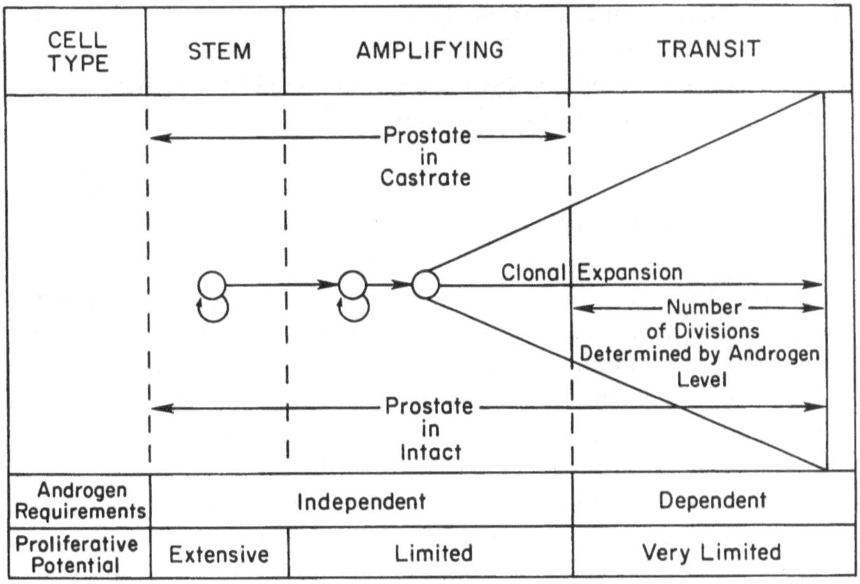

Fig. 1 Stem Cell Model for the Organization of the Prostate
Stem cells are androgen-sensitive during the development of their full number. Once the total stem cell number is reached, stem cells become androgen-independent.

and still fully restore the gland. These results demonstrated that both stem cells and amplifying cells are able to maintain themselves (i. e. renew themselves) during long term androgen withdrawal (i. e. they are androgen-independent). This androgen independence does not mean, however, that these cells are completely insensitive to androgenic stimulation, only that they do not absolutely require such androgenic stimulation for their continuous maintenance. As discussed earlier, there are cells within the prostate of an intact adult host which do absolutely require a critical level of androgen stimulation for their continuous presence since these cells are rapidly eliminated from the gland following castration (i. e. they are androgen-dependent). These cells, termed transit cells, are derived from the pool of amplifying cells (fig. 1). Once such a transit cell is produced it can proliferate only a limited number of times. The total number of proliferations (i. e. population doublings) of these transit cells is determined by the level of androgenic stimulation within certain physiologic limits as discussed previously. The androgen-stimulated clonal expansion of these transit cells eventually results in the prostate growing to its maximal normal size. In reaching this maximal size, the transit cells quantitatively become the vast majority of cells present in the prostate. For this reason, the total prostatic cell number is highly androgen-sensitive since following castration the rate of cell death of these transit cells is much higher than their rate of cell proliferation and therefore these transit cells are rapidly eliminated from the prostate. Since these transit cells are the vast majority of cells present in the normal prostate, their elimination leads to the rapid prostatic involution even though the stem cells and the amplifying cells are still maintained following castration.

What causes BPH?

Based upon the stem cell model presented in Figure 1 for the organization of prostate, there are at least two distinct ways in which BPH could theoretically develop from the normal prostate. Since each prostatic stem cell subserves a hierarchically expanding population of amplifying cells, which in turn subserves an expanding population of transit cells, an increase in total stem cell numbers would directly result in enlarged prostates. Alternatively, since both the amplifying and transit cells are capable of limited clonal expansion, as defined by the maximum number of population doublings each can undergo before senescence, an abnormal increase in this clonal expansion number can also produce an enlarged prostate. At present, it is unknown which of these two alternatives or both is involved in BPH. In order to clarify this important issue, some understanding as to what normally controls the total number of stem cells present within the prostate and what determines the clonal expansion number from the amplifying and transit cells is urgently needed.

What controls the total number of stem cells present within the prostate

For both the rat and dog, the total number of stem cells within the prostate is effected by material released from the testes. This was first demonstrated by the observation of Rajfer and Coffey [29] that if male rats are castrated between birth and 50 days of age and allowed to go untreated until reaching adulthood (i. e. 70 days of age) before being subsequently treated with exogeneous androgen, the prostate only grows to 40 – 50% of its normal adult size no matter how high a replacement dose of androgen is used [11, 29]. These earlier observations have been repeated to test the effect of castration at different ages on the subsequent response of the rat ventral prostate to exogeneous androgen. To do this, animals were castrated at either 20, 50, or 90 days of life and left either untreated or implanted with a 2.5 cm long testosterone filled silastic capsule per rat at the time of castration or 40 days following castration. The size of testosterone implant was chosen to restore the serum testosterone level to a value of 2 – 3 ng/ml, which is identical to physiological level observed in intact controls. After 1

Table 1 Effect of castration at different ages and the subsequent response of the rat ventral prostate to exogeneous testosterone

Age at Castration DAYS	Age at Testosterone Replacement[a] (DAYS)	Ventral Prostatic Cell Number at 1 year of Age
Non-castrated	–	16.8 ± 0.9 (100%)[b]
20	–	0.95 ± 0.05 (5.6%)
20	20	17.2 ± 1.5 (102%)
20	60	6.72 ± 0.50 (40%)
50	–	1.25 ± 0.04 (7.4%)
50	50	16.2 ± 1.1 (96%)
50	90	15.4 ± 1.2 (92%)
90	–	1.12 ± 0.09 (6.7%)
90	90	17.0 ± 0.8 (101%)
90	130	15.8 ± 1.2 (94%)

[a] A 2.5 cm long testosterone filled silastic capsule was implanted S. Q. in each rat. This size implant restored the serum testosterone level to the physiological levels in intact normal rate (i. e. 2 – 3 ng/ml).

[b] Values in parentheses are the percentage vs the non-castrated animals.

year of treatment, the total number of ventral prostatic cells was determined for each rat (table 1). These results demonstrated that if sufficient androgen is not chronically maintained up to 50 days of life in the rat, then it is not possible to stimulate the full development of the involuted prostate to reach its maximum normal size at 1 year of life. In additional studies, rats were castrated at 20 days of life and implanted with two 2.5 cm long testosterone filled implants which are able to elevate the serum testosterone more than two-fold above normal (i. e. >6 ng/ml) and these rats were followed-up to 1 year of treatment, however, again the ventral prostate cell number was still only 41% of that of 1 year old intact control rats. In direct contrast to these findings, if adequate androgen is present up to day 50 of life, however, it is possible to remove the testes and allow the prostate to involute and then treat with androgen 40 days later and still fully restore the normal size of the prostate at 1 year. These results suggest that with rat ~ 60% of the total ventral prostatic stem cells are produced between 20 and 50 days of life and that at least a portion of the prostate stem cells are dependent upon androgen for their initial development. A similar observation is also true for the dog. If beagles are castrated at 14 months of age and allowed to go untreated for an additional 46 months (i. e. until 5 years of age) and then treated for 6 months with exogeneous testosterone and estradiol filled silastic implants which restore the normal physiological level of this steroid in the blood, the involuted prostate grows to only ~ 50% of size of the prostate of age matched (i. e. 66 months old) beagles never castrated [13]. In contrast, if 2 year old beagles are castrated and allowed to go untreated for 5 months, and then given the same testosterone and estradiol treatment for 7 months, the involuted prostate grow to 100% of size of the prostate of age matched beagles never castrated [4].

These combined results demonstrate that in the rat the total stem cell number is reached by 50 days of life (i. e. 5% of total life-span) while in the dog, the total number of stem cells is not reached in a normal gland until 2 years of age (i. e. 20% of total life). In both species, however, the initial development of the total normal number of stem cells is androgen responsive. In the rat once the number of prostatic stem cells is reached, this number becomes androgen-independent. This is demonstrated by the fact that if rats are castrated at 50 days of age and allowed to go untreated for 1 year before being treated with physiological levels of androgen, it is possible to fully restore the total cell number of these prostates within one month of treatment to the identical value obtained from 1 year old intact male rats never castrated. If 20 or 50 day old rats are not castrated but instead given pharmacologically high doses of androgen, the prostate increases its normal growth rate by two-fold. By twenty days of treatment, the total number of ventral prostate cells reach the maximal value normal serum only after 1 year in an untreated control rat. Whereas the rate at which the maximal cell number is reached is greatly increased by pharmacologically high levels of androgen, continuous exposure to high level of androgen, even for more than 600 days is not able to increase the total prostatic cell number above what is observed for 1 year old untreated male rats [6]. These results demonstrate that during the initial period of up to 50 days of life in the rat, the total number of stem cells is reached and that during this period the initial development of this number depends on a certain level of androgenic stimulation. Once this critical level of androgenic stimulation (i. e. physiological levels of androgen) is reached, further increases in androgenic stimulation (i. e. pharmacological level of androgen) can not induce an overgrowth of stem cells to produce an abnormally enlarged gland.

The situation for the dog is quite different. While the development of the normal number of stem cells likewise minimally requires a physiological level of androgen during a critical period (i. e. up to 2 years of life), pharmacologically high levels of androgen can induce the abnormal increase in stem cell number. This is demonstrated by the fact that young dogs (2–3 years old) can be induced to develop a greater than 2-fold abnormal overgrowth of the prostate (i. e. BPH development) simply by treatment with high levels of androgen with a small amount of estradiol [12, 31]. Whether a similar treatment with high levels of androgen could likewise induce precociously the development of prostatic overgrowth (i. e. BPH development) in young adult human males is unknown. It is

Table 2 Prostatic growth rates in the rat, dog and human under a variety of conditions

Species	Growth Rate (Expressed as Prostatic Volume Doubling Time in Days) During				
	Development of gland to a normal adult size[a]	Restoration of adult gland following castration induced involution[b]	Spontaneous development of BPH	Restoration of BPH following androgen ablation induced involution[c]	Maximum androgen stimulation of intact host[d]
Rat	12	5	–	–	5
Dog	233	14	334	14	40
Man	1015	?	931	292	?

[a] For rat, determined between 20–70 days of age [6]; for dog, determined between 1 and 24 months of age [7]; for human, determined between 10–20 years of life [8, 20].

[b] For rat, 1 year old animals were castrated and allowed to involute for 1 month, then restored with physiological levels of androgen [6]; for the dog, two year old animals were castrated and 5 months of involute, then restored with physiological levels of androgen [4].

[c] For dog, 6–8 year old dogs with spontaneous BPH were castrated and allowed to involute for 5 months, then treated with physiological levels of androgen [4]; for human, patients were treated with LHRH analog for 6 months, then treatment was stopped [28].

[d] For rat, 50 day old rats were treated with pharmacologically high levels of androgen [6]; for dog, 2–3 year old dogs were treated with pharmacologically high levels of androgen plus estradiol [12].

known for both the dog and man, however, that once BPH develops in an intact host it is possible to cause an involution of the BPH tissue by means of androgen ablation [4, 28]. In addition, if after a period of involution, normal physiologic levels of androgen are restored the BPH tissue is fully restored to its abnormal size in both species [4, 28].

A comparison of the prostate growth rates in rat, dog, and human under a variety of conditions, table 2 suggests fundamental differences in these species. For the rat, the growth rate during restoration of the involuted gland in a castrated adult and the maximal rate of growth driven by pharmacological androgen stimulation are equal and more than two-fold faster than the growth rate during the normal development of adult gland. This again demonstrates that maximal number of prostate stem cells are already present in the rat by 50 days of life and that while pharmacological androgen can increase the growth rate (i. e. for 12 to 5 days doubling time), it can not induce any abnormal increase in total stem cell number. For the dog, the growth rate during restoration of either the normal adult gland or BPH gland induced to involute following castration, is equal and is nearly 3-fold faster than the rate of maximally androgen-stimulated growth during BPH development and more than 15-fold greater than the growth rate during development of the normal adult prostate. This suggests that during both the normal glandular development and BPH development, the number of stem cells present is the rate limiting factor in determining the rate of prostatic growth and that this number is slowly increasing to a maximum with time. Once this maximum number is reached in the normal gland (i. e. by 2 years of age), it is possible to allow the prostate to involute and then fully restore the gland with physiological androgen at a much faster growth rate (i. e. 14 day doubling time) than seen during the initial growth of gland to its normal adult size (i. e. 233 day doubling time).

This is because now the only limitation to the rate of growth is the rate at which the amplifying and transit cells can clonally expand. Similar, once the total number of stem cells is reached in BPH (i. e. this number is abnormally higher in BPH than that in normal gland), it is possible to allow the BPH tissue to involute and then fully restore the gland with physiological androgen at a much faster growth rate than seen during the spontaneous development of BPH. Again, this probably is due to the fact that this restoration growth only requires clonal expansion of the amplifying and transit cells without any requirement for prostatic stem number to increase. This restoration rate of growth is nearly threefold higher than the growth rate during maximum androgen stimulation of intact adult dogs during the experimental induction of BPH by pharmacologically high level of androgen. This suggests that such pharmacologically high levels of androgen stimulation of intact adult dogs induces not only the clonal explansion of the amplifying and transit cells but also the increase in prostate stem cell number.

While all of the comparable human growth rate data are not available, it is known that the growth rate during the early development of the normal adult prostate [20] is approximately equal to the growth rate of spontaneous BPH development [21]. The rate of restoration of human BPH, induced to involute by 6 months of LHRH treatment, is however more than 3-fold faster than either of these other rates [7] (Table 2). This again suggests that during the spontaneous development of BPH in human the number of stem cells must increase as well as the total number of amplifying and transit cells.

Is BPH due just to an increase in total stem cell number?

While the preceding discussion clearly suggests that in BPH of both dog and man there is an abnormal increase in total stem cell number with increasing aging, is this increase in stem cell number alone responsible for BPH? The answer to this question is probably *no* for both dog and man. If BPH was due to simply an increase in the total number of prostate stem cells, then while the BPH gland would be abnormally enlarged, BPH tissue should be phenotypically equivalent to normal non-BPH prostatic tissue. Comparison of the biochemistry of normal and BPH tissue in humans and dogs have demonstrated clear differences between these tissues. These changes include differences in androgen metabolism [10, 18, 22, 23], androgen receptor content [1, 30], degree of methylation of the cytosine residues in the DNA [2] and secretory protein (e. g. acid phosphotase) [10]. These phenotypic differences suggest that not only the number of stem cells is increased in BPH as compared to the normal gland, but also the ratio between stem, amplifying and transit cells is also changed. This would mean that there are differences in the clonal explansion number as well as differences in the number of stem cells present in BPH.

References

[1] Barrack, P., P. C. Walsh: Subcellular distribution of androgen receptors in human normal, benign hyperplastic, and malignant prostatic tissues: Characterization of nuclear salt-resistant receptors. Cancer Res. *43* (1983) 1107 – 1116.

[2] Bedford, M. T., P. D. van Helden: Hypomethylation of DNA in pathological conditions of the human prostate. Cancer Res. *47* (1987) 5274 – 5276.

[3] Berg, O. A.: Parenchymatous hypertrophy of the canine prostate gland. Acta Endocrinol. *27* (1952) 140 – 154.

[4] Berry, S. J., D. S. Coffey, J. D. Strandberg et al.: Effect of age, castration, and testosterone replacement on the development and restoration of canine benign prostatic hyperplasia. The Prostate *9* (1986) 295 – 302.

[5] Berry, S. J., D. S. Coffey, P. C. Walsh et al.: The development of human benign prostate hyperplasia with age. The Journal of Urology *132* (1984) 474.

[6] Berry, S. J., J. T. Isaacs: Comparative aspect of prostatic growth and androgen metabolism with aging in the dog versus the rat. Endocrinol. *114* (1984) 511 – 520.

[7] Berry, S. J., J. D. Strandberg, W. J. Saunders et al.: Development of canine benign prostatic hyperplasia with age. The Prostate *9* (1986) 363 – 373.

[8] Boyd, E.: Growth, including reproduction and morphological development. In: D. Altman (ed.): Biological Handbooks, Federation of American Societies for Experimental Biology, pp. 346 – 348. Washington, D. C. 1962.

[9] Brendler, C. B., S. J. Berry, L. L. Ewing et al.: Spontaneous benign prostatic hyperplasia in the beagle: Age-associated changes in serum hormone levels and morphology and secretory function of the canine prostate. J. Clin. Invest. *71* (1983) 1114 – 1123.

[10] Brendler, C. B., A. L. Follansbee, J. T. Isaacs: Discrimination between normal, hyperplastic and malignant human prostatic tissues by enzymatic profiles. The Journal of Urology *133* (1985) 495.

[11] Chung, L. W., D. K. MacFadden: Sex steroids imprinting and prostatic growth. Investigative Urology *17* (1980) 337.

[12] DeKlerk, D. P., D. S. Coffey, L. L. Ewing et al.: Comparison of spontaneous and experimentally induced canine prostatic hyperplasia. J. Clin. Invest. *64* (1979) 842.

[13] Ewing, L. L., D. S. Coffey, J. Strandberg et al.: (Unpublished data) 1988.

[14] Goldstein, S., C. B. Harley, E. J. Moerman: Some aspects of cellular aging. J. Chron. Dis. *36* (1983) 103 – 116.

[15] Hayflick, L.: Recent advances in the cell biology of aging. Mechanism of Aging and Development *14* (1980) 59–79.
[16] Huggins, C.: The etiology of benign prostatic hypertrophy. Bull. NY Acad. Med. *23* (1947) 696.
[17] Huggins, C., P. J. Clark: Quantitative studies of prostatic secretion II. The effect of castration and of estrogen injection on the normal and on the hyperplastic prostate glands of dogs. J. Exp. Med. 72 (1940) 747–762.
[18] Isaacs, J. T.: Changes in dihydrotestosterone metabolism and the development of benign prostatic hyperplasia in the aging beagle. J. Steroid Biochem. *18* (1983) 749.
[19] Isaacs, J. T.: Antagonistic effect of androgen on prostatic cell death. The Prostate *5* (1984) 545–557.
[20] Isaacs, J. T.: Common characteristics of human and canine benign prostatic hyperplasia. In: F. A. Kimball, A. E. Buhl, D. B. Carter (eds): New Approaches to the Study of Benign Prostatic Hyperplasia, p. 217. Alan R. Liss Co., New York 1984.
[21] Isaacs, J. T.: Control of cell proliferation and cell death in the normal and neoplastic prostate: A stem cell model. In: C. H. Rodgers, D. S. Coffey, G. Cunha (eds): Benign Prostatic Hyperplasia, pp. 85–94. U. S. Dept. of Health and Human Services, NIH Publication #87–2881, 1987.
[22] Isaacs, J. T., C. B. Brendler, P. C. Walsh: Changes in the metabolism of dihydrotestosterone in the hyperplastic human prostate. J. Clin. endocrinol. Metabol. *56* (1983) 139.
[23] Isaacs, J. T., D. S. Coffey: Changes in dihydrotestosterone metabolism associated with the development of canine benign prostatic hyperplasia. Endocrinol. *108* (1981) 445.
[24] Isaacs, J. T.: (Unpublished data) 1988.
[25] Kyprianou, N., J. T. Isaacs: Quantal relationship between prostatic dihydrotestosterone and prostatic cell content: Critical threshold concept. The Prostate *11* (1987) 41–50.
[26] Lesser, B., N. Bruchovsky: The effects of 5α-dihydrotestosterone in the kinetics of cell proliferation in rat prostate. Biochem. J. *142* (1974) 483–489.
[27] Moore, R. A.: Benign hypertrophy and carcinoma of the prostate. In: G. Twombly, G. Packs (eds): Endocrinology of Neoplastic Diseases, pp. 194. Oxford Press, London – New York 1947.
[28] Peters, C. A., P. C. Walsh: The effect of nafarelin acetate, a luteinizing-hormone-releasing hormone agonist, on benign prostatic hyperplasia. N. Engl. J. Med. *317* (1987) 599–604.
[29] Rajfer, J., D. S. Coffey: Sex steroid imprinting of the immature prostate: Long-term effect. Investigative Urology *16* (1978) 186.
[30] Trachtenberg, J., L. L. Hicks, P. C. Walsh: Androgen- and estrogen-receptor content in spontaneous and experimentally induced canine prostatic hyperplasia. J. Clin. Invest. *65* (1980) 1051–1059.
[31] Walsh, P. C., J. D. Wilson: The induction of prostatic hypertrophy in the dog with androstanediol. J. Clin. Invest. *57* (1976) 1093.
[32] Zukerman, S., T. McKeown: The canine prostate in relation to normal and abnormal testicular changes. J. Pathol. Bacteriol. *46* (1938) 7–19.

Benign prostatic hyperplasia: morphometric studies in relation to the pathogenesis*

G. Bartsch, A. Brüngger, U. Schweikert, H. Hintner, R. Höpfl, H. P. Rohr

Morphological approach

The histology of the normal human prostate and the histopathology of benign prostatic hyperplasia have been well documented [6, 7, 11, 12, 18, 19, 21, 22]. The possible role of stromal tissue in the pathogenesis of benign prostatic hyperplasia was for the first time suggested in 1925 [23]; the initial lesions of benign prostatic hyperplasia were apparently fibromyomatous nodules into which penetration of glandular elements occured. In order to be able to establish a structure-function relationship, these morphological methods were complemented by quantitative techniques which yield objective and reproducible values for any morphological structure thus allowing statistical comparisons. This can be achieved by stereological methods.

Stereology, a term coined by the International Society in 1961, is based on geometric probability and makes it possible to quantitate three-dimensional structures by extrapolation from measurements of two-dimensional cross-sections thereof. Further methodological details (calculations, multistage sampling were described by Weibel and Rohr [24].

Light microscopic findings

To evaluate the prostatic gland and its components in stereological terms a morphometric model of the human prostate was developed [1, 2, 24]. Figure 1 shows how the human prostate was divided into morphologically defined compartments. Essentially the model has two major divisions – the stromal part (ST) including connective tissue, blood vessels, nerves and smooth muscle fibres and the glandular part (EP) including the lumina of the acini and the glandular epithelial cells.

* Supported by the Fonds zur Förderung der wissenschaftlichen Forschung (P 4020) Austria and the Swiss National Foundation No. 3190 – 0.82.

New Developments in Biosciences 5

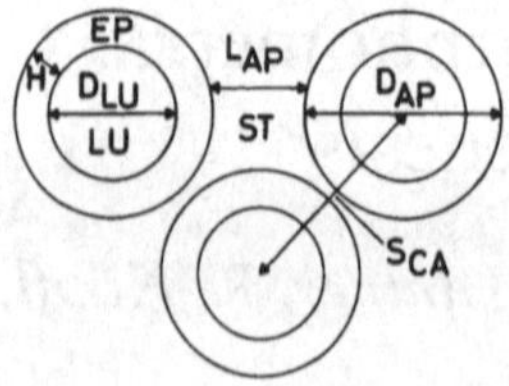

Fig. 1 Stereological model of the human prostate.

The following absolute stereologic parameters were determined:

Surface density of the glandular epithelium (S)
Volume density of the stromal part (V_{ST})
Volume density of the epithelial part (V_{EP})
Volume density of the glandular lumen (V_{LU})
Length density of the glandular tubules (L)
Height of the glandular epithelium (H)
Diameter of the glandular lumen (D_{LU})
Diameter of the glandular tubules (D_{AP})
Mean free distance between the glandular tubules (L_{AP})
Mean distance between the centers of the glandular tubules (S_{CA}).

As can be seen from the absolute data (table 1) in benign prostatic hyperplasia in comparison to normal prostatic tissue there is a statistically significant increase in the volumetric amount of stromal tissue and the glandular lumina; contrary, regarding the volumetric amount of glandular epithelium no difference between normal and hyperplastic tissue can be found; there is also no difference regarding the surface density and the height of epithelial cells; as a consequence of the highly significant increase in stromal tissue a significant increase in the mean free distance between the glandular tubules (= L_{AP}) and the mean distance between the centers of the glandular tubules (= S_{CA}) was found in hyperplastic tissue.

Ultrastructural findings

The smooth muscle cells in the normal human prostate are spindle-shaped. Most of the organelles are located near the nucleus or in small clusters in the cell periphery. Most of the cytoplasm is occupied by myofilaments. The rough endoplasmic reticulum consists of a few profiles of membranes, a great part of which is often devoid of ribosomes; sometimes a small Golgi apparatus and few mitochondria can be observed. Contrary to these findings, in benign prostatic hyperplasia the perinuclear zone is markedly increased. The abundant rough

Table 1 Absolute data of normal and hyperplastic prostatic tissue

Stereologic analysis	case	age	weight (g m)	S $\times 10^5$ mm^2	V_{LU} $\times 10^3$ mm^3	V_{EP} $\times 10^3$ mm^3	V_{ST} $\times 10^3$ mm^3	L $\times 10^5$ mm	H u	D_{LU} u	D_{AP} u	L_{AP} u	S_{CA} u
Hyperplastic	1	80	87	7.63	43.2	12.9	31.4	18.3	17	226	260	199	459
	2	72	42	2.58	8.7	4.9	28.4	8.1	19	134	173	479	652
	3	63	36	2.98	8.9	4.9	22.3	7.4	16	120	153	332	485
	4	52	79	5.96	14.5	11.7	52.6	15.0	20	97	137	392	529
	5	73	62	3.32	7.0	7.9	46.9	13.9	24	84	132	613	745
	6	76	204	17.90	78.6	29.1	97.0	50.0	16	176	208	249	457
	7	72	42	34.60	13.5	6.4	22.6	11.4	19	156	193	298	492
	8	79	56	3.92	16.7	6.4	33.8	13.2	16	170	203	378	581
	9	71	50	3.49	13.9	7.5	28.6	12.1	22	159	202	371	574
	10	62	84	1.94	10.9	3.4	16.1	5.6	18	225	261	368	629
	m ± SD	71 ± 9	74 ± 49	8.4 ± 10.3	21.5 ± 22.5	9.5 ± 7.4	37.9 ± 23.5	15.5 ± 12.7	18.7 ± 2.7	154.7 ± 47.9	192.2 ± 45.1	367.9 ± 116.4	560.3 ± 94.3
Normal	1	24	19	2.30	5.32	4.23	6.7	7.9	18	93	129	152	382
	2	26	24	3.17	6.78	7.38	10.2	5.1	23	85	132	176	308
	3	21	22	2.49	5.57	4.55	9.6	5.5	18	89	126	190	316
	m ± SD	23 ± 2	21.6 ± 2.5	2.6 ± 0.4	5.8 ± 0.7	5.3 ± 1.7	8.8 ± 1.8	6.1 ± 1.5	19.6 ± 2.8	89.0 ± 4.0	129.0 ± 3.0	172.6 ± 19.2	335.3 ± 40.6

endoplasmic reticulum shows enlarged cisternae studded with ribosomes. The Golgi apparatus is also enlarged and contains more vesical than cisternal elements [3, 25].

Data for the various smooth muscle cell compartments are given in table 2. In benign prostatic hyperplasia there is a statistically significant increase in the volume fractions of rough endoplasmic reticulum, mitochondria and Golgi apparatus.

Table 2 Volume densities of smooth muscle cells in the normal human prostate and benign prostatic hyperplasia

	Golgi apparatus*	Organelles*	Myofilaments*
Normal human prostate, 5 pts.			
Mean	0.002	0.048	0.950
Standard error	0.001	0.005	0.026
Benign prostatic hyperplasia, 5 pts.			
Mean	0.013	0.134	0.853
Standard error	0.001	0.006	0.032

* Analysis of variance-significant.

These light and electron microscopic measurements show that tissue overgrowth in human benign prostatic hyperplasia is mostly due to an increase in stromal tissue; as shown by the electron microscopic measurements, in the benign prostatic hyperplasia-changed prostatic tissue activated smooth muscle cells are observed, which possibly play a key role in the pathogenesis of human benign prostatic hyperplasia.

Correlation of stereological and biochemical results

Since the initial studies of Siiteri and Wilson in 1970 [31] it has become apparent that alterations in androgen metabolism are responsible for the spontaneous development of human benign prostatic hyperplasia. However, supranormal 5α-dihydrotestosterone levels were not found in hyperplastic human prostatic tissue most recently by Walsh [32]. At present there are strong indications that it is above all androgens which control the function of the stromal part of the human prostate; therefore, an attempt was made to correlate the quantitative morphologic and biochemical values of normal and hyperplastic prostatic tissue to find out, if this altered steroid metabolism in benign prostatic hyperplasia is reflected in the morphologic architecture.

Endogenous hormone analyses

Benign prostatic hyperplasia tissue specimens were obtained by means of open prostatectomy; normal prostatic tissue was obtained from kidney donors.

Extraction of steroids: 1 g of tissue was homogenized in 2 ml of ethanol with an Ultra Turrax. The homogenizer was washed with 2 ml of cold ether which were then added to the homogenate. The extraction was performed overnight by vertical rotation of the tubes containing the homogenate. After centrifugation the supernatant was transferred to a second tube and the pellet was washed with 4 ml of ether. Then the supernatant was again centrifuged and added to the first one. The combined extracts were dried up with a stream of nitrogen. The residue was dissolved in 2 ml of methanol and water (volume 90/10) and extracted with 5 ml of petrol ether. 2 ml of water were added to the methanol ether layer and the mixture was extracted three times with 2 ml of ether. Finally, the combined ether extracts were dried up with nitrogen. The recovery was 70% for testosterone, 69% for 5α-dihydrotestosterone, 85% for estrone, 89% for estradiol and 93% for estriol.

Radioimmunoassay: Testosterone and 5α-dihydrotestosterone were separated and purified with the help of celite microcolumns and then measured by radioimmunoassay; E 1, E 2, and E 3 were separated on sephadex LH 20 columns according to Edquist and Johansson (1972). E 1 and E 2 were analyzed by radioimmunoassay with the help of an antiserum which reacts with estrone and estradiol to the same extent; the E 3 radioimmunoassay was performed by employing a specific estriol antiserum.

Regarding the endogenous tissue levels no significant difference was found between the estrone, estradiol, estriol (table 3) and progesterone (table 4) levels of normal and hyperplastic tissue. The endogenous concentrations of 5α-dihydrotestosterone and testosterone were examined in 10 patients with BPH and in five normal prostates, in which a stereologic analysis was also performed. In addition the endogenous testosterone and 5α-dihydrotestosterone concentrations were examined in another 15 samples of BPH. No statistically significant difference was found between normal and hyperplastic tissue (normal tissue: 4.2 $\pm$ 0.7 ng/ml, BPH: 10 specimens: 7.0 $\pm$ 2.9 ng/ml, BPH: 15 specimens: 4.1 $\pm$ 0.7 ng/ml, table 5, 6).

By using the Spearman rank correlation coefficient a statistical analysis was performed for age, weight of the prostate, absolute stereologic results and the following biochemical data: endogenous prostatic hormones (5α-dihydrotestosterone, testosterone, progesterone, estradiol, estrone and estriol) (table 7).

Table 3 Endogenous estrone, estradiol and estriol tissue levels in the normal and hyperplastic human prostate

	case	age	weight (gm)	tissue levels estrone (ng/gm)	estradiol (ng/gm)	estriol (ng/gm)
Hyperplastic	1	80	87	0.90	0.05	0.03
	2	72	42	0.14	0.06	0.02
	3	63	36	0.12	0.06	0.02
	4	52	79	0.08	0.03	0.02
	5	73	62	0.07	0.06	0.02
	6	76	204	0.13	0.07	0.03
	7	72	42	0.04	0.04	0.04
	8	79	56	0.12	0.06	0.02
	9	71	50	0.09	0.04	0.02
	10	62	84	0.14	0.11	0.03
	m ± SD	71 ± 9	74 ± 49	0.10 ± 0.03	0.06 ± 0.02	0.02 ± 0.01
Normal	1	24	19	0.19	0.03	0.02
	2	26	24	0.13	0.03	0.02
	3	21	22	0.10	0.06	0.07
	m ± SD	23 ± 2	21.6 ± 2.5	0.14 ± 0.04	0.04 ± 0.02	0.04 ± 0.03

Table 4 Endogenous progesteron tissue levels in the normal and hyperplastic human prostate

	case	age	weight (gm)	tissue level progesterone (ng/gm)
Hyperplastic	1	80	87	0.770
	2	72	42	0.074
	3	63	36	0.055
	4	52	79	0.050
	5	73	62	0.083
	6	76	204	0.055
	7	72	42	0.048
	8	79	56	0.048
	9	71	50	0.036
	10	62	84	0.040
	m ± SD	71 ± 9	74 ± 49	0.059 ± 0.022
Normal	1	24	19	0.055
	2	26	24	0.065
	3	21	22	0.063
	m ± SD	23 ± 2	21.6 ± 2.5	0.061 ± 0.005

Table 5 Endogenous testosterone and 5α-dihydrotestosterone tissue levels in the normal and hyperplastic human prostate

	case	age	weight (gm)	tissue levels testosterone (ng/gm)	dihydrotestosterone (ng/gm)
Hyperplastic	1	80	87	0.21	8.0
	2	72	42	0.36	5.2
	3	63	36	0.33	3.6
	4	52	79	0.29	6.5
	5	73	62	0.85	7.5
	6	76	204	0.91	8.0
	7	72	42	0.94	8.5
	8	79	56	0.45	3.9
	9	71	50	0.95	13.8
	10	62	84	1.60	5.1
	m ± SD	71 ± 9	74 ± 49	0.69 ± 0.44	7.0 ± 2.9
Normal	1	24	19	0.17	2.9
	2	26	24	0.14	1.5
	3	21	22	0.21	3.2
	m ± SD	23 ± 2	21.6 ± 2.5	0.17 ± 0.03	2.5 ± 0.9

Table 6 Endogenous 5α-dihydrotestosterone tissue levels in hyperplastic prostatic human tissue

	case	age	weight (gm)	tissue levels testosterone (ng/gm)	dihydrotestosterone (ng/gm)
Hyperplastic	1	72	67.4	0.21	4.4
	2	74	31.6	0.31	3.5
	3	82	83.8	0.16	5.1
	4	68	70.0	0.20	4.0
	5	63	97.2	0.30	3.8
	6	76	42.1	0.30	3.6
	7	78	85.1	0.60	5.1
	8	83	102.2	0.30	4.7
	9	77	79.4	0.30	4.7
	10	75	73.2	0.70	3.5
	11	73	116.2	2.80	3.6
	12	72	123.4	1.40	4.4
	13	82	92.0	0.90	4.8
	14	69	25.7	0.70	5.4
	15	73	36.1	0.20	4.4
	m ± SD	74 ± 5	75.0 ± 30.1	0.75 ± 0.75	4.3 ± 0.6

Table 7 Correlation of age, weight of the prostate, biochemical and absolute stereological data

	Age	weight	V_{LU}	V_{EP}	V_{ST}	S	L	H	D_{LU}	D_{AP}	L_{AP}	S_{CA}
Testosterone										○		○
5α-dihydrotestosterone	○	●	○	○	○	○	●			○		○
Estradiol												
Estrone												
Estriol												
Progesterone												
Androgen Receptor (N)					○						○	
Androgen Receptor (C)												
Estrogen Receptor (N)												
Estrogen Receptor (C)												
Progesterone Receptor (C)			○						○	○		

● $p < 0.01$ N: Nucleus
○ $p < 0.05$ C: Cytoplasm
All other values do not show a statistically significant correlation

As it can be seen from the statistical analysis no statistically significant correlation coefficient was obtained for the endogenous 5α-dihydrotestosterone concentration and the age of the patient as well as the weight of the prostate; a statistically significant correlation (weak) could only be found for the glandular tissue and the surface density of glandular epithelium. The estriol, estradiol, estrone and endogenous progesterone steroid levels did not correlate significantly with the morphometric data investigated; these data show that stromal overgrowth in benign prostatic hyperplasia does not correlate with the endogenous androgen, estrogen and progesterone levels.

This study shows that prostatic overgrowth in the aging male is only poorly reflected in the endogenous hormone levels of the whole prostate. Thus, in order to clarify the etiology of this disease, other factors must be studied. Factors of the extracellular matrix, which possibly control the growth and function of the glandular epithelium, should be investigated in future studies; on the other side the high amount of secretory products in large BPH samples should be investigated with regard to neurotransmitters.

Hormone sensitivity of stromal tissue

There is some evidence that interactions between stromal and epithelial cells play a crucial role in the regulation of the coordinated growth of the prostatic gland. Since the separation of prostatic acinar parenchyma and stroma is difficult or even impossible and in common biochemical practice prostatic tissue is homogenized prior to biochemical assays, most biochemists overlooked the cellular elements of the stromal tissue. Therefore the stromal function regarding hormonal response is virtually not understood. Despite the fact that receptor proteins have been found for estrogens, testosterone and 5α-dihydrotestosterone the action site of these steroids in the different glandular and stromal cell components has not been demonstrated. Thus the role of glandular and stromal elements of the prostate in steroid metabolism is still unclear.

It was shown that the endogenous concentration of 17β-estradiol in the stromal part of the prostate of guinea pigs exceeded those of blood plasma and prostatic epithelium; this fact supports the assumption that endogenous estrogen may play a role in the regulation of male accessory sex tissue and smooth muscle cell function [5]; an activation of the smooth muscle cells of the uterus of prepubertal rats was demonstrated after injection of 17β-estradiol [29]. In young female virgin mice estrogen injections for 3 days led to an increase in the cell organelles of the smooth muscle cells of the uterus [26]. These autoradiographic findings show that under definite experimental conditions the smooth muscle cells can participate in the synthesis of ground substance of connective tissue. In strong a/J strain mice enlargement of the prostate and the periurethral gland can be produced by estrogens [10].

Similar results of smooth muscle cell activation were obtained in beagle dogs following estrogen administration, which indicates that possibly estrogens play a role in the induction of stromal growth by smooth muscle cell activation [27]. In relation to the unit volume of smooth muscle cell cytoplasm, in castrated dogs treated with estrogens (2.5 mg of estradiolbenzoate twice a week over a period of 3 weeks) a statistically significant increase in the volume of rough endoplasmic reticulum, vacuoles and vesicles can be seen compared to the control group [27]. These stereological results are very similar to those obtained for smooth muscle cells in human benign prostatic hyperplasia. These data possibly reemphasize the fact that estrogens play a role in the development of human benign prostatic hyperplasia.

A precise understanding of the estrogenic action at the cellular level of human benign prostatic hyperplasia and in particular on the stroma is still lacking. An important supposition for discussing specific estrogenic action is the demonstration of estrogens in human benign prostatic hyperplastic tissue. When comparing stroma to the epithelium in human benign prostatic hyperplasia Krieg et al. found an accumulation of estrogens in the nuclei of stromal cells [16]. Krieg et al. furthermore showed in the stromal cells more estrogen receptor positive cases than in the epithelial cells [16]. These data possibly support the hypothesis that 17β-estradiol plays a special role in stimulating the growth of the stromal part of the human prostate.

At present there are strong indications that it is above all androgens which control the function of the stromal part of the human prostate. In 1977 Cowan and coworkers for the first time reported that 5α-reductase activity, which regulates 5α-dihydrotestosterone formation, was found predominantly in the stromal tissue of the prostate [9]. Using a mechanical technique for separating the glandular and stromal parts Krieg, Romijn and Bruchovsky [8, 15, 28] found that 5α-reductase activity in the stromal fraction of the prostate was considerably higher than in the glandular fraction; by comparing the stromal fractions of the normal human prostate and benign prostatic hyperplasia it was shown that the mean specific activity of 5α-reductase in benign prostatic hyperplasia is three times greater [8].

The 5α-reductase and 3α(β)-hydroxysteroid oxidoreductase activity of the stromal and glandular parts in the normal human prostate and in benign prostatic hyperplasia were analyzed without the use of these separation techniques which possibly destroy the cell architecture and the stromal/glandular interrelationships. In a correlative biochemical and light microscopic stereological study testosterone metabolite formation was measured in small biopsy specimens; afterwards a stereological analysis was performed to determine the amounts of glandular and stromal tissue [30].

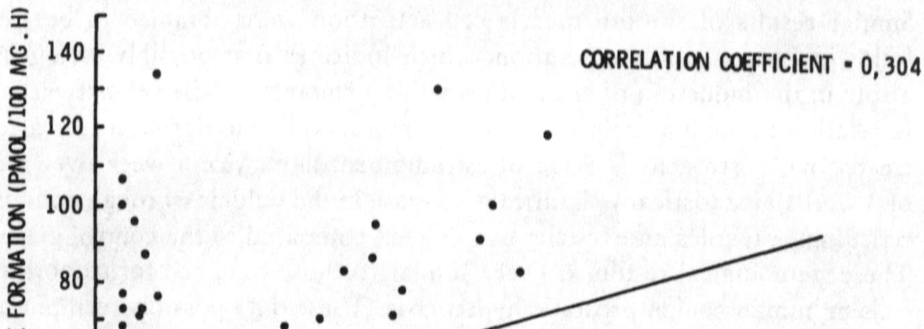

Fig. 2 Correlative biochemical and morphometric study on human biopsy specimens, 5α-reductase activity is correlated to the amount for stromal and glandular tissue of the biopsy specimen (= 100%), hyperplastic prostatic tissue.

As can be seen from the correlation coefficient there is no difference between 5α-dihydrotestosterone and 5α-androstane 3α(β)17β-diol formation when the testosterone metabolism of the stromal part is compared to that of the glandular part (fig. 2 and 3). These data on intact tissue show that 5α-reductase and 3α(β)-hydroxysteroid oxidoreductase activity is found in benign prostatic hyperplasia in the stromal part as well as in the glandular part.

The discrepancy of these values may be due to the methods employed. It is understandable that mechanical separation disturbs the integrity of the cells, in particular of the more vulnerable epithelial cells, which in turn may affect the cellular metabolism. The advantage of the method employed in this study over the methods in which the stromal and glandular parts are separated mechanically is that the tissue used for assessing the metabolic rates is left intact.

Summarizing the results of these biochemical and morphological investigations on the hormone responsiveness of prostatic stromal tissue one can say that stromal tissue is possibly sensitive to both estrogens and androgens: regarding androgen metabolism these investigations also show that stroma is not only a target tissue but also an active metabolizing component in the prostate.

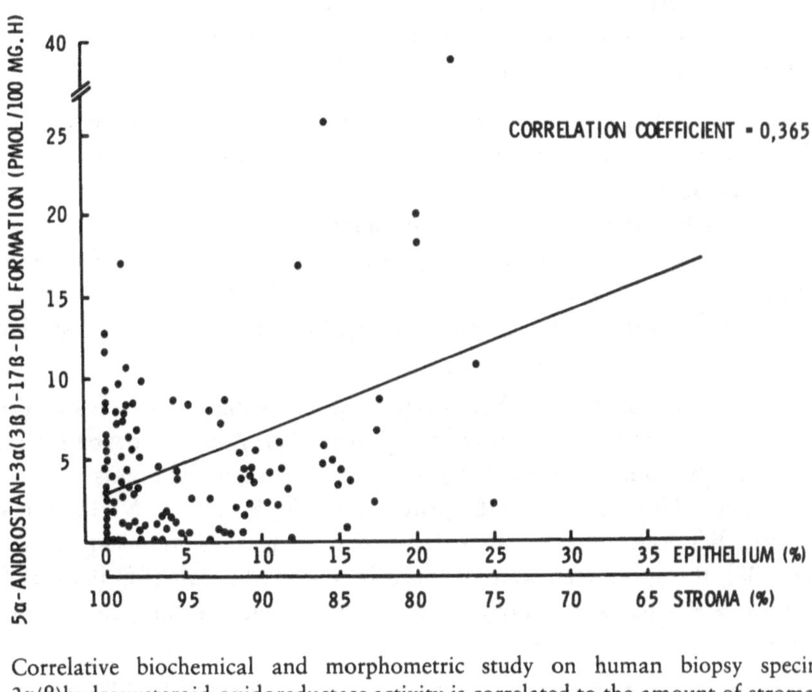

Fig. 3 Correlative biochemical and morphometric study on human biopsy specimens, 3α(β)hydroxysteroid-oxidoreductase activity is correlated to the amount of stromal and glandular tissue of the biopsy specimen (= 100%), hyperplastic prostatic tissue.

Extracellular matrix

There is strong evidence that the extracellular matrix acts as an interface between epithelial and stromal cell elements, such as smooth muscle cells and fibroblasts; although the exact nature and composition of the extracellular matrix in the prostate, is not known at present, in most tissues it is composed of collagen, glycosaminoglycans and glycoproteins. Glycosaminoglycans were shown to play an important role in the development and growth of normal and neoplastic tissue. As compared to the normal human prostate, increased levels of chondroitin sulphate were shown in benign prostatic hyperplasia [14]. It was shown that this interface plays an important role in glandular-stromal interactions as well as in the development of the normal prostate and in benign prostatic hyperplasia. The biochemical mechanism of these interactions remains obscure; however, the understanding of the mechanism of the interface and the influence of ageing and hormonal alterations on this factor will be of great help in the understanding of the pathogenesis of benign prostatic hyperplasia.

Numerous studies performed over the past decade support the concept that smooth muscle cells are multifunctional cells capable of synthesizing collagen, elastin, myosin and glycosaminglycans. It was demonstrated in cultures that in vitro these smooth muscle cells can synthesize type I and III collagens [17]. On the other hand smooth muscle cells were shown to be involved also in the process of collagen phagocytosis and degradation [13].

Previous studies have shown that type I and III collagens comprise the major fibrillar protein components found in the connective tissue of skin, blood vessels and stromal tissue of visceral organs. Other types of collagen are restricted to hyaline cartilage (type II) and basement membrane (type IV). The purpose of the present study was to investigate the presence and distribution of various types of collagen (type I, III and V) and laminin, a non-collagenous basement membrane glycoprotein found in the normal human prostate and in benign prostatic hyperplasia.

Cryostat sections of normal human (n = 3) or benign hyperplastic prostates (n = 5) were first incubated, for thirty minutes with rabbit antitype I, III and IV collagen serum (concentration: 1 : 80) or with rabbit anti-laminin serum (concentration: 1 : 40). All sera were kindly provided by Dr. S. J. Katz, National Institutes of Health, Bethesda, Maryland. After extensive washes in phosphate-buffered saline (PBS), the specimens were exposed in a second incubation period of thirty minutes to a fluorescin isothiocyanate- (FITC) labelled swine anti-rabbit serum of a dilution of 1 : 20.

In a control group these specific antisera were substituted by PBS or by a non-immune rabbit serum during the first incubation period. A cryostat section of a normal human prostate, which was incubated with PBS and afterwards with FITC-labelled swine anti-rabbit serum served as a negative control; beside the very faint background there was no specific staining, neither in the epithelium nor in the stromal part of the specimen.

Specific immunofluorescence staining of sections of normal human and hyperplastic prostates with rabbit antibodies against type I collagen was observed only within the stromal tissue, whereas the glandular cells remained completely unstained. Note that antibodies against type I collagen in the normal prostate (fig. 4) stain strongly and appear as bundles around a group of smooth muscle cells, whereas among the individual smooth muscle cells only faint staining can be observed.

In benign prostatic hyperplasia, due to the stromal overgrowth, this typical scaffold pattern is replaced by a strong, diffuse distribution of the antibody reactivity (fig. 5).

Very similar to type I collagen, the antibody reactivity of collagen type III was present only within the stromal tissue, whereas the glandular cells remained unstained. Individual or grouped smooth muscle cells are interwoven with delicate type III positive fibres originating from a scaffold of thick, coarse collagen

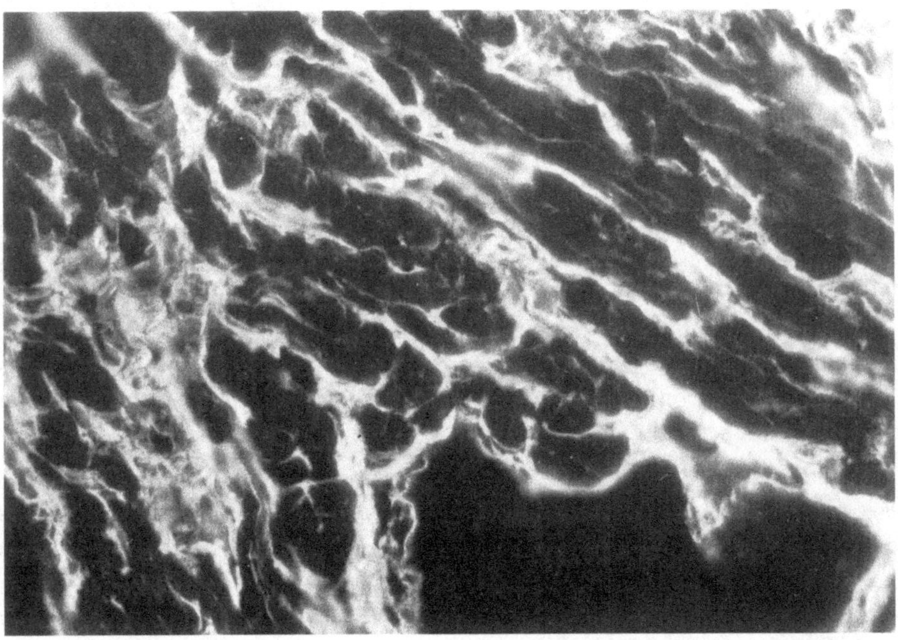

Fig. 4 Collagen type I: specific immunofluorescence staining of sections of normal human prostatic tissue.

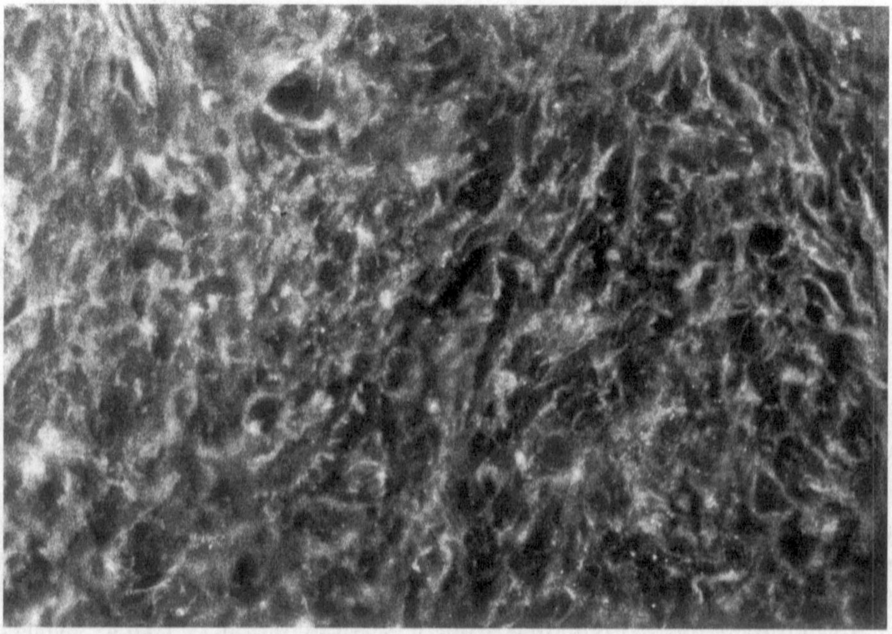

Fig. 5 Collagen type III: specific immunofluorescence staining of sections of hyperplastic prostatic tissue.

bundless in normal prostatic tissue. In benign prostatic hyperplasia this subtle architecture is replaced by a dense array of irregularly interlaced wavy type III collagen fibers between the stromal cells (= fibroblasts, smooth muscle cells).

Contrary to type I and III collagen the fluorescence staining of type IV collagen in normal as well as in benign prostatic hyperplasia tissue was found to outline smooth muscle cells in a regular honey-comb pattern; due to the increase in stromal tissue in benign prostatic hyperplasia a more irregular pattern of type IV collagen immunofluorescence was observed in benign prostatic hyperplasia; nevertheless, the antibody reactivity was found to outline only the stromal cells in a regular honey-comb pattern; as regards the immunofluorescence staining with antilaminin serum the same picture as with type IV collagen antiserum was observed.

These studies suggest a considerable overproduction of type I and III collagens in benign prostatic hyperplasia, which demonstrates that these two collagens are principal factors in the stromal character of human benign prostatic hyperplasia; whether the overproduction of collagen observed is the cause or the result of the stromal function has to be elucidated in future studies.

Stromal induction using strong a/J mice subjected to long-term treatment with estrogen

In 1933 and 1966, respectively, Lacassagne as well as Fingerhut and Veenema [10] described another valuable model applicable for research on benign prostatic hyperplasia. Lacassagne injected an oily solution of estrogen once a week, whereas Fingerhut and Veenema used strong a/J mice, who were treated by subcutaneous implantation of pellets containing diethylstilbestrol. After several months, both authors described the occurrence of urinary retention evoked by compression of the urethra or the bladder neck, and metaplastic changes of the prostatic epithelium. Fingerhut and Veenema also mentioned an enlarged stromal compartment around the bladder neck, in which whorl-like nodules occurred [10].

Sexually mature intact a/J mice were treated by subcutaneous injections of 0.1 mg of estradiol valerianate; after 12 weeks of treatment the animals were sacrificed and the accessory sex glands, the bladder neck and the bladder excised simultaneously, weighed and submitted to histologic and electron-microscopic processing.

After treatment with estradiol two main alterations can be observed: 1. regions with an increased amount of fibromuscular tissue, 2. some acini with metaplastic processes of the glandular epithelium. Not all parts of the prostatic complex show the same degree of stromal growth, which is most extensive in the region of bladder neck.

Two types of fibromuscular stroma can be distinguished: 1. tightly packed smooth muscle cells forming rings around the prostatic acini, 2. very loose interstitial tissue filling the space between the basal membrane of the glandular epithelium and the surrounding rings of the smooth muscle cells of an acinus (fig. 6). Sometimes the increase in the fibromuscular stroma results in the formation of whorl-like nodules or slings.

The fibromuscular stroma reveals fibrocytes, smooth muscle cells, macrophages and sometimes a very loose interstitial tissue containing only few fibrocytes and smooth muscle cells (fig. 7). In the estrogen-treated animals the smooth muscle cells are often intensively activated. This activation manifests itself in increased amounts of cytoplasmic organelles – preferably in the perinuclear region – a nucleus with many infoldings and marked vesicular activity along the cellular membrane (fig. 8). The onset of metaplastic processes can easily be detected on account of an increased number of desmosomes and bundles of tonofilaments as well as decreased secretory activity.

The stromal reaction pattern of the a/J mice is of great interest, especially because of the bladder neck obstruction which occurs in connection with stromal overgrowth. It is interesting that the fibromuscular stroma of the prostatic complex

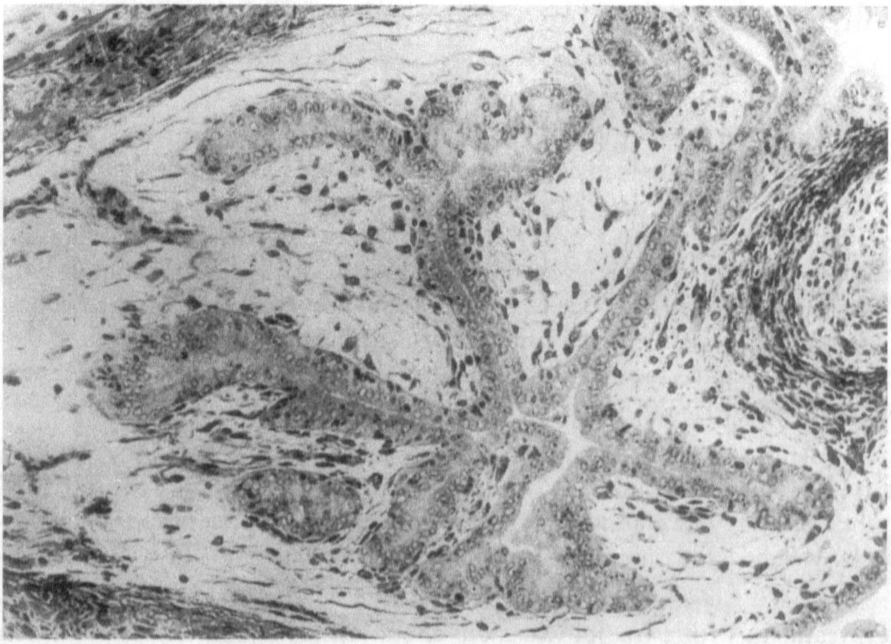

Fig. 6 Tightly packed smooth muscle cells forming rings around the prostatic glands.

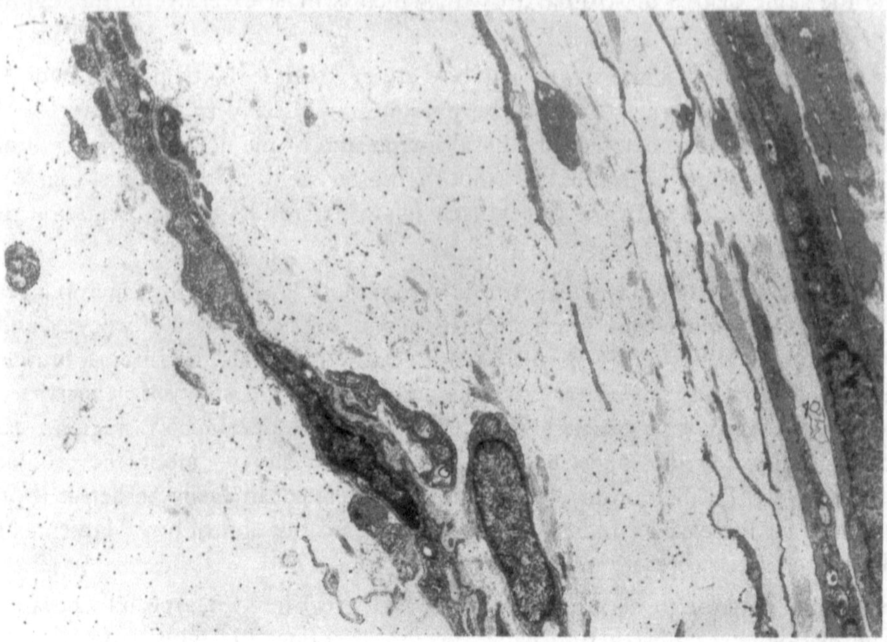

Fig. 7 Loose interstitial tissue containing only few fibrocytes and smooth muscle cells.

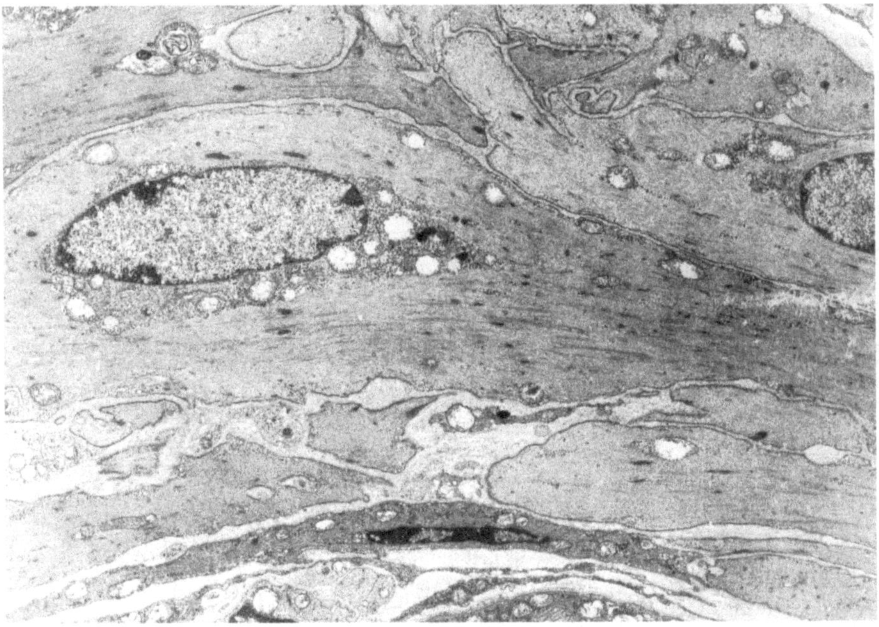

Fig. 8 Activated smooth muscle cells in estrogens-treated animals with increased amounts of cytoplasmic organelles.

does not react homogeneously to estrogen stimulation; if the fibromascular stroma proliferates and forms whorl-like nodules, squamous metaplasia of the glandular cells, especially in the coagulation glands, can be observed. These findings show that there is even focally a great interaction between stromal and epithelial cell elements. This is possibly one explanation for the hyperplastic alterations of the prostate as it was assumed in human benign prostatic hyperplasia by McNeal in 1978 [20].

Further studies will have to find out whether collagen synthesis is hormone-sensitive; we furthermore will have to study collagen degradation and find out whether type I or III collagen synthesis in hyperplastic tissue is reversible by hormonal manipulation.

References

[1] Bartsch, G., E. Fischer, H. P. Rohr: Ultrastructural morphometric analysis of the rat prostate (ventral lobe). Urol. Res. *3* (1975) 1.

[2] Bartsch, G., H. P. Rohr: Ultrastructural stereology: a new approach to the study of prostatic function. Invest. Urol. *14* (1977) 301 – 306.

[3] Bartsch, G., J. Frick, I. Ruegg et al.: Electron microscopic stereological analysis of the normal human prostate and of benign prostatic hyperplasia. J. Urol. *122* (1979) 481–486.

[4] Bartsch, G., H. R. Müller, M. Oberholzer et al.: Light microscopic stereological analysis of the normal human prostate and of benign prostate hyperplasia. J. Urol. *122* (1979) 487–491.

[5] Blume, D. C. H., M. G. Mawhinney: Estrophilic molecules in the male guniea-pig. J. Steroid Biochem. *9* (1978) 515–529.

[6] Brandes, D.: Fine structure and cytochemistry of male sex accessory organs. In: D. Brandes (ed.): Male Accessory Sex Organs: Structure and Function in Mammals. pp. 18–44. Academic Press, New York 1974.

[7] Brandes, D., D. Kirchheim, W. Scott: Ultrastructure of the human prostate: normal and neoplastic. Lab. Invest. *13* (1964) 1541.

[8] Bruchovsky, N., T. Callaway, G. Lieskovsky et al.: Markers of androgen action in human prostate: potential use in the clinical assessment of prostatic carcinoma. In: J. L. Witliff, O. Dapunt (eds): Steroid Receptors and Hormone Dependent Neoplasia, pp. 121–132. Masson, USA 1980.

[9] Cowan, R. A., S. K. Cowan, J. K. Grant et al.: Biochemical investigations of separated epithelium and stroma from benign prostatic hyperplastic tissue. J. Endocr. *14* (1977) 111–116.

[10] Fingerhut, B., R. J. Veenema: Histology and radioautography of induced benign enlargement of the mouse prostate. Invest. Urol. *4* (1966) 112–124.

[11] Franks, L. M.: Benign nodular hyperplasia of the prostate: a review. Ann. Roy. Coll. Surg., Engl. *14* (1954) 92.

[12] Franks, L. M.: Benign prostatic hyperplasia: gross and microscopic anatomy. In: J. T. Grayhack, J. D. Wilson, M. J. Scherbenske (eds): Benign Prostatic Hyperplasia. National Institute of Arthritis, Metabolism and Digestive Disease, Workshop Proceedings, pp. 63–89. Bethesda 1975.

[13] Jurukova, Z., Ch. Milenkov: Involvement of smooth muscle cells in collagen degradation in the postpartum uterus. Virchows Arch. *37* (1981) 237–244.

[14] DeKlerk, D. P.: Glycosaminoglycans of benign prostatic hyperplasia. American Urological Association, Kansas City 1982.

[15] Krieg, M., G. Klötzl, J. Kaufmann et al.: Stroma of human benign prostatic hyperplasia: perferential tissue for androgen metabolism and estrogen binding. Acta Endocr., Copenh. *96* (1981) 422–432.

[16] Krieg, M., W. Bartsch, M. Thomsen et al.: Androgens and estrogens: Their interaction with stroma and epithelium of human benign prostatic hyperplasia and normal prostate. J. Steroid. Biochem *19* (1983) 155–161.

[17] Layman, D. L., E. H. Epstein, Jr., R. F. Dodson et al.: Biosynthesis of type 1 and 3 collagens by cultured smooth muscle cells from human aorta. Proc. Natl. Acad. Sci. *74* (1977) 671–675.

[18] Mao, P., K. Nakao, R. Bora et al.: Human benign prostatic hyperplasia. Arch. Path. *79* (1965) 270.

[19] McNeal, J. E.: Development and comparative anatomy of the prostate. In: J. T. Grayhack, J. D. Wilson, M. J. Scherbenske (eds): Benign Prostatic Hyperplasia. National Institute of Arthritis, Metabolism and Digestive Disease, Workshop Proceedings, pp. 1–9. Bethesda 1975.

[20] McNeal, J. E.: Origin and evolution of benign prostatic enlargement. Invest. Urol. *15* (1978) 340.

[21] Moore, R. A.: Benign hypertrophy of the prostate. A morphological study. J. Urol. *50* (1943) 680.

[22] Narbaith, R.: Embryology, anatomy and histology of the male sex accessory glands. In: D. Brandes (ed.): Male Accessory Sex Organs: Structure and Function in Mammals, pp. 3–15. Academic Press, New York 1974.

[23] Reischauer, F.: Die Entstehung der sogenannten Prostatahypertrophie. Virch. Archiv 256 (1925) 357–389.

[24] Rohr, H. P., M. Obholzer, G. Bartsch et al.: Morphometry in experimental pathology (Methods, baseline, data and applications) Int. Rev. Exp. Pathol. *15* (1976) 233–325.

[25] Rohr, H. P., G. Bartsch: Human benign prostatic hyperplasia: a stromal disease. New perspectives by quantitative morphology. Urology (1980) 625–633.

[26] Rohr, H. P., Z. Jurukova: Beiträge zur Bildung bindegewebiger Matrix in glatten Muskelzellen. Path. Eur. *3* (1978) 571–592.

[27] Rohr, H. P., H. F. Naef, O. Holliger et al.: The effect of estrogen and stromal growth of the dog prostate. Urol. Res. *9* (1981) 201–207.

[28] Romijn, J. C., K. Oishi, J. Belt de Vries et al.: Androgen metabolism and androgen receptors in separated epithelium and stroma of the human prostate. In: F. H. Schröder, H. J. de Voogt (eds): On Steroid Receptors, Metabolism and Prostatic Cancer, pp. 134–139. Excerpta Medica, Amsterdam 1980.

[29] Ross, R., S. J. Klebanoff: Fine structural changes in uterine smooth muscle and fibroblasts in response to estrogen. J. Cell. Biol. *32* (1967) 155–159.

[30] Schweikert, H. U., G. Bartsch, P. Totzauer et al.: Testosterone metabolism in the epithelium and stroma of normal human prostate in benign prostatic hyperplasia. (In press, 1983).

[31] Siiteri, P. K., J. D. Wilson: Dihydrotestosterone in Prostatic Hypertrophy. I. The Formation and Content of Dihydrotestosterone in the Hypertrophic Prostate of Man. J. Clin. Invest. *49* (1970) 1737–1745.

[32] Walsh, P. C.: Human benign prostatic hyperplasia: Etiological considerations. In: F.-A. Kimball, A. E. Buhl, D. B. Carter (eds): New Approaches to the Study of Benign Prostatic Hyperplasia, pp. 1–25. Alan R. Liss, Inc., New York 1984.

The extracellular matrix and cellular proliferation in the etiology of benign prostatic hyperplasia

M. Mawhinney

Microanatomy

Male accessory sex organs, including the prostate gland, are composed of two tissues, the epithelium and smooth muscle, separated by the connective tissue interface or the lamina propria. These three components are readily visible with the light microscope. At low power electron microscopy, the epithelial tissue is composed of a single layer of tall columnar secretory epithelial cells along with a small number of basal cells resting on the basal lamina, collectively termed the basement membrane. One of the lamina, the lamina lucida or rara, is represented by the clear zone immediately under the epithelial cells, while the other adjoining deeper layer is an electron dense band termed the lamina densa, and borders on the lamina propria. Proteoglycans are the primary constituents of the lamina lucida, and are large aggregates of protein coupled with glycosaminoglycans (acid mucopolysaccharides), which are polymers of a repeating unit of sulfated and acetylated amino hexoses and uronic acids. Deklerk [7] has measured the content of the glycosaminoglycans in isolated epithelial cell fractions obtained through use of a Latapie press. Due to the requisites of the isolation procedure, the integrity of the basal lamina was uncertain, but the fraction was free of collagen. The epithelial fraction contained chrondroitin sulfates A & C and dermatan sulfate. No heparan sulfate was found and only 2.5% of the total pool was hyaluronic acid. The lamina densa consists primarily of type IV collagen, which is organized into a mesh or network [18] rather than the fibrillar structure commonly associated with interstitial collagens, such as types I & III. Connective tissue glycoproteins, including laminin and fibronectin, may serve to physically and functionally integrate the cell membrane and the basal lamina [12]. Recently, receptors for these connective tissue glycoproteins have been identified [13, 26], and are termed integrins. Integrins represent a family of receptor proteins, which have in common a recognition site for the tri-peptide sequence arginine-glycine-aspartic acid commonly found in connective tissue glycoproteins and collagens. Although multiple integrins have been identified, it appears that fibronectin and laminin act and interact at the same receptor molecule in the extracellular space [14]. Integrins are transmembrane molecules with the intracellular component

New Developments in Biosciences 5

interacting with actin filaments and having a site subject to modulation by phosphorylation [13, 26]. An additional development potentially relevant to understanding the epithelial cell extracellular matrix is the identification of type VII collagen, which may form anchoring fibrils [2]. While not yet identified in the prostate gland, anchoring fibrils may serve to bind the lamina densa to the underlying lamina propria.

The epithelial cell basal lamina are produced primarily, if not completely, by the epithelial cells, and are the object of much research into the potential role in supporting or regulating normal and neoplastic cellular functions. As a part of this regulation, the lamina may provide a physical barrier and biochemically modulate [10] the blood born factors to epithelial cells, since capillaries are confined to the lamina propria side of the basal lamina.

In muscle tissue, muscle cells are imbedded in a connective tissue matrix, although the lamina surrounding the smooth muscle cells do not appear in a clear layered fashion [11]. Proteoglycans and type IV collagen can be found in close association with muscle cell membranes along with the glycoproteins, fibronectin, laminin, and thrombospondin [12, 28]. At the present time, little has been accomplished to identify these matrix components and their functional significance in male accessory sex organ smooth muscle. Muscle interstitium or the connective tissue between muscle cells is the region where fibrillar collagens such as types I, III, and the associated type V are found along with the proteoglycans and glycoproteins.

Smooth muscle in BPH

Benign prostatic hyperplasia (BPH) can be viewed as a new organ developing from the internal or peri-urethral portions of the prostate gland between the bladder neck and the verumontanum. In the fully developed state, the ratio of the muscle tissue or fibromuscular stroma to epithelium is 5 : 1, which is significantly greater than the normal peripheral prostate gland [24]. However, it is unknown at the present time whether the ratio of these two tissues in the neoplasm is abnormal relative to the site(s) of origin. Within the periurethral regions of the prostate gland, the initial cell types involved in the proliferative response appear to be either fibroblasts or smooth muscle cells of the sub-mucosal glands (peri-urethral glands or glands of Albarran) or peri-urethral smooth muscle. Specifically, in 1939, LeDuc [17] confirmed observations of Albarran and Halle in 1900 and of Reischauer in 1925, that the first detectable proliferative response appeared in spindle shaped cells with a paucity of smooth muscle fibers relative to smooth muscle cells located in the inter-acinar stroma of normal prostate glands. The observation was also made that such fibroblast appearing cells involved in the proliferative response in the developing nodule appeared to have de-differentiated to lose muscle fibers. In the same year, Deming and Wolfe [8] reported the initial lesion in BPH was a fibromuscular mass in the urethral smooth muscle, but whether the cells involved resembled fibroblasts or smooth muscle cells was not determined. Moore [20], in 1943 identified that either fibroblasts or smooth muscle cells may be the origin of the initial growth. A peri-urethral cell consistent with the morphology of a fibroblast was also reported by Pradhan and Chandra [23] to be the origin of BPH. McNeal [19] identified two cell types and sites of origin for small lesions less than 3 mm.

First, those in the peri-urethral smooth muscle were fibroblastic, and secondly, those in the newly defined transition zone, which borders on the outer aspect of the urethral smooth muscle, were of epithelial cell origin. Finally, it should be recognized that Frank's [19] research led to the conclusion that the initial cell type of origin could not be stated with certainty, and that epithelial cell or stromal cell hyperplasia could occur alone or together. Therefore, based on the majority of reports, the fibromuscular stroma is of key significance in BPH, representing the primary mass in the fully developed adenoma, as well as its site of origin, with either fibroblasts or smooth muscle cells in the peri-urethral glands or sphincteric smooth muscle being the cells involved in the initial proliferative response.

Although the etiology of the renewed proliferation of either fibroblasts or smooth muscle cells in the peri-urethral zone of the prostate gland is not known at the present time, several mechanisms can be reasonably proposed. The epithelium of the developed adenoma is primarily columnar, but about 20% of the nodular epithelium can be classed as inactive with resemblance to pre-pubertal cells or adult cells receiving minimal androgenic stimulation [20]. In addition, a declining viability of acinar epithelium in the true prostate gland was reported as a universal finding in all prostates developing BPH [ibd.]. As reviewed by LeDuc [17] Albarran and Halle actually reported that very early fibrous nodules developed around remnants of glandular structures, but this has not been confirmed.

Given the observations of some degree of reduced epithelial cell viability in adenomas in association with developing adenomas, it should be noted that the etiology of fibromuscular proliferation in arterioles has been traced to endothelial cell damage and removal of the anti-proliferative glycosaminoglycan layer between endothelial cells and smooth muscle tissue [28]. Heparin and structurally related glycosaminoglycans have been shown to inhibit smooth muscle cells proliferation in vitro and in vivo [3]. Such findings raise the possibility that one of the initial triggers for focal fibroblast and/or smooth muscle cell growth in BPH may be traced to reduced inhibitory effect of extracellular matrix molecules secondary to a declining or altered production by less viable epithelial cells.

Proliferation of mesenchymally derived cell types may involve a transient change in phenotype, and support through autocrine mechanisms, particularly the production of platlet derived growth factor (PDGF). As previously noted, proliferating fibroblast-like cells de-differentiated from muscle cells, based on the presence of muscle fiber remnants [17]. As adenomas developed in size, more poorly differentiated stromal cells differentiated into the smooth muscle phenotype [20]. It is notable that the perinuclear region of muscle cells from BPH is rich in organelles [24]. In relation to normal prostate muscle, muscle cells from BPH have an approximate 6-fold increase in the volume density of the Golgi apparatus, and an approximate 3-fold increase in the total organelle volume density which includes Golgi, rough endoplasmic reticulum and mitochondria, coupled with a slight decrease in myofilaments. The potential importance of these observations eminate from numerous lines of evidence obtained from aortic smooth muscle showing that proliferating smooth muscle cells exhibit a secretory or synthetic phenotype (increased ratio of organelles to myofilaments). Primary muscle cell cultures plated at relatively low density revert from the contractile to synthetic phenotype and proliferate in response to serum or PDGF [27]. Specific morphological features of these proliferating cells include increases in both the rough endoplasmic reticulum and free ribosomes, and decreases in desmin, alpha actin, and myofilaments relative to contractile cells, findings which are consistent with the phenotype of the muscle cell from the aortic wall during its proliferative phase in young animals [ibd.]. Such a synthetic phenotype of abundant cytoplasmic organelles is also observed in the proliferating muscle tissue adjacent to atherosclerotic plaques [21], and in the estrogen-induced growth of the myometrium [25]. The conditioned medium from primary cultures of proliferating muscle cells induced proliferation in growth arrested secondary cultures [22]. The medium competed for PDGF binding and its mitogenic activity was neutralized by a PDGF antibody. Seifert et al. [29] compared PDGF production by cultured young and adult muscle cells and found the young to produce as much as 1000 X more mitogen. Experiments with a smooth muscle tumor cell line, which was initially derived by the combined testosterone propionate and diethylstiebestrol-induction of a leiomyosarcoma in hamster vas deferens, have shown that androgens stimulate cell growth, while glucocorticoids are antagonistic involving PDGF as an intermediate [30]. Glucocorticoids inhibit the production of transcripts (m-RNA) homologous to v-sis and the blockade of proliferation can be surmounted by the addition of PDGF or conditioned medium from cells not exposed to glucocorticoid. The other potentially significant mesenchymal mitigen now known to exist in the prostate gland is basic fibroblast growth factor (FGF) [31]. Having recently identified this mitogen in the prostate gland, it will be of particular interest to determine the level of FGF as well as PDGF expression around the initial proliferations in the peri-urethral zone known to represent the origins of the disease.

Epithelial tissue in BPH

Since the early 1900's, renewed growth of the epithelium in BPH has been viewed as a consequence of the inductive influence of the proliferating fibromuscular stroma. Although no evidence presently exists to directly support the idea that adult smooth muscle tissue regulates growth of epithelium, embryonic urogenital mesenchyme induces normal embryonic epithelial morphogenesis [6]. Chungs's research [5] with embryonic inductors has found that adult mouse prostate gland growth was increased 10- to 20-fold by intra-prostatic implantation of intact embryonic urogenital sinus. Growth of the organ system was due in part to actual regrowth of the host prostate. Separation of the embryonic urogenital sinus into epithelial and mesenchynial components with subsequent implantation into adult hosts revealed that the isolated tissues were much less active than inact urogenital sinus; only the mesenchyme retained some degree of inductive activity. In view of the observations that either proliferating fibroblasts or smooth muscle cells represent the initial lesion in BPH, it may ultimately be possible to develop experimental systems, along the lines of the Chung model system, to duplicate some of the concepts of tissue-tissue interactions by implanting populations of cultured prostatic fibroblasts, smooth muscle cells, or extracellular components into normal host organs of experimental animals.

Within the epithelial tissue, evidence has accrued in a variety of systems to demonstrate the significance of the basal lamina, particularly type IV collagen, in epithelial cell proliferation and differentiation. Mammary gland epithelial cells synthesize and deposit type IV collagen in culture, which supports both cellular attachment and proliferation [35]. In regressed ventral prostate from adult castrated rats, dihydrotesterone (DHT) increased total collagen synthesis as early as day one of treatment, an effect which was increased and sustained for 7 days [33]. During this time frame, there was not only an approximate three-fold increase in DNA, but a major transition in cellular differentiation from cuboidal non-secretory cells to a tall columnar secretory epithelium. Total collagen levels, however, did not increase until day 7, indicating that during the early phase of androgen-induced growth, collagen degradation balanced synthesis. In estrogen-induced rat uterine growth, plasminogen activator, a potential activator of collagenase, increased 12 hours prior to the onset of DNA synthesis [16]. This potential turnover of collagens appears to be important to support the androgen-induced growth, since cis-hydroxyproline (CHP) treatment, which inhibits collagen degradation and perturbed epithelial basal lamina inhibited both the proliferation and normal differentiation of epithelial cells [33]. Based on research with the MCF-7 mammary cell line and with melanoma cells, the cellular interaction with and metabolism of basement membranes is controlled in part by laminin and fibronectin. In cultured MCF-7 cells, estrogen treatment enhanced cellular migratrion through polycarbonate membranes coated with type IV collagen to laminin but not fibronectin [1]. By direct measurement of type IV collagenase activity in a melanoma cell line, it was likewise demonstrated that laminin was stimulatory, but fibronectin had no effect [34]. However, fibronectin had the potential to block collagenase activity possibly by inhibiting laminin binding. There were also in vivo correlates of these experiments in that laminin or fibronectin treatment of melanoma cells in culture caused a respective stimulation or inhibition of invasion in vivo [32]. Therefore, since these two glycoproteins appear to act through the same integrin molecule [14], the relative increase in production of laminin vs. fibronectin during the early androgen-induced growth response may be a requisite for initiating basement membrane remodeling.

The transition from proliferation to maintenance of maximal levels of fully differentiated prostatic epithelium may involve cessation of active basement remodeling and activation of processes supportive of terminal differentiation. Various epithelial chalones including TGF-beta [4] may be involved in maintenance of the non-proliferative differentiated state, but no well defined mechanisms have yet been elucidated for the prostate gland. TGF-beta has been shown to be anti-proliferative for epithelial cells, and two of its characteristic effects are the stimulation of fibronectin and collagen type I production [15]. Possibly transition to the non-proliferative state involves inhibition of further basement membrane remodeling by increased fibronectin and development of the connective tissue outerface between epithelium and muscle. Should this prove correct, deficient production or sensitivity to such chalones may be of etiological significance in BPH.

Summary

The development of BPH represents a multifaced problem consistent with that of organogenesis. It potentially involves stimulatory and inhibitory interactions between epithelium and smooth muscle tissues, as well as a dynamic interplay between the cells of each tissue and the associated extracellular matrix. Our understanding of this disease can be significantly enhanced by focusing attention on model systems, which allow for resolution of specific components of these different processes at specific stages of cellular and tissue growth. Understanding the mechanism for the reawakened proliferation of peri-urethral fibroblasts or smooth muscle cells is central to our understanding of the etiology of this adenoma.

References

[1] Albini, A., J. Graf, G. T. Kitten et al.: 17 B-Estradiol regulates and v-Ha-ras transfection constitutively enhances MCF7 breast cancer cell interactions with basement membrane. Proc. Natl. Acad. Sci. *83* (1986) 8182–8186.

[2] Burgeson, R. E., N. P. Morris, L. W. Murray et al.: The structures of type VII Collagen. Annals New York Academy Sciences *469* (1985) 47–57.

[3] Castellot, J. J., J. Choay, J.-C. Lormeau et al.: Structural determinants of the capacity of heparin to inhibit the proliferation of vascular smooth muscle cells. II. Evidence for a pentasaccharide sequence that contains a 3-O-sulfate group. J. Cell Biol. *102* (1986) 1979–1984.

[4] Cheifetz, S., J. A. Weatherbee, M. L. S. Tsang et al.: The transforming growth factor-beta system, a complex pattern of cross-reactive ligands and receptors. Cell *48* (1987) 409–415.

[5] Chung, L. W. K., J. Matsuura, M. R. Runner: Tissue interactions and prostatic growth. I. induction of adult mouse prostatic hyperplasia by fetal urogenital sinus implants. Biol. of Repro. *31* (1984) 155–163.

[6] Cunha, G. R., L. W. K. Chung, J. M. Shannon et al.: Stromal-epithelial interactions in sex differentiation. Biol. of Repro. *22* (1980) 19–41.

[7] DeKlerk, D. P.: The glycosaminoglycans of normal hyperplastic prostate. Prostate *4* (1983) 73–81.

[8] Deming, C. L., J. S. Wolf: the anatomical origin of benign prostatic enlargement. J. Urology *42* (1939) 566–580.

[9] Franks, L. M.: Benign prostatic hyperplasia; gross and microscopical anatomy. In: J. Grayhack, J. Wilson, M. S. Scherbenske (eds): Benign Prostatic Hyperplasia, pp. 63–90. DHEW publication (NIH) 76–1113, Bethesda 1975.

[10] Gordon, M. Y., G. P. Riley, S. M. Watt et al.: Compartmentalization of a haematopoietic growth factor (GM-CSF) by glycosaminoglycans in the bone marrow microenvironment. Nature *326* (1987) 403–405.

[11] Hascall, V. C., G. K. Hascall: Proteoglycans. In: E. Hay et al. (ed.): Cell biology of the extracellular matrix, pp. 39–64. Plenum Press, New York 1981.

[12] Haynes, R. O.: Fibronectin and its relation to cellular structure and behavior. In: E. Hay et al. (ed.): Biology of the extracellular matrix, pp. 295–334. Plenum Press, New York 1981.

[13] Haynes, R. O.: Integrins: A family of cell surface receptors. Cell *48* (1987) 549–554.

[14] Horwitz, A., K. Duggan, R. Greggs et al.: The cell substrate attachment (CSAT) antigen has properties of a receptor for laminin and fibronectin. J. Cell Bio. *101* (1985) 2134–2144.

[15] Ignotz, R. A., J. Massague: Cell adhesion protein receptors as targets for transforming growth factor-Beta action. Cell *51* (1987) 189–197.

[16] Kneifel, M. A., S. P. Leytus, E. Fletcher et al.: Uterine plasminogen activator activity: modulation by steroid Hormones. Endocrinology *111* (1982) 493–499.

[17] LeDuc, I. E.: The anatomy of the prostate and the pathology of early benign hypertrophy. J. Urology *42* (1939) 1217–1241.

[18] Mayne, R.: Collagenous proteins of blood vessels. Arteriosclerosis *6* (1986) 585–593.

[19] McNeal, J. E.: Origin and evolution of benign prostatic enlargement. Inves. Urol. *15* (1978) 340–345.

[20] Moore, R. A.: Benign hypertrophy of the prostate. J. Urology *50* (1943) 680–709.

[21] Mosse, P. R., G. R. Campbell, Z. L. Wang et al.: Smooth muscle phenotypic expression in human carotid arteries I. Comparison of cells from diffuse intimal thickenings adjacent to atheromatous plaques with those of the media. Lab. Inves. *53* (1985) 556–562.

[22] Nilsson, J., M. Sjolund, L. Palmberg et al.: Arterial smooth muscle cells in primary culture produce a platlet derived growth factor like protein. PNAS *82* (1985) 4418–4422.
[23] Pradhan, B. K., K. Chandra: Morphogenesis of nodular hyperplasia-prostate. J. Urology *113* (1975) 210–213.
[24] Rohr, H. P., G. Bartsch: Human benign prostatic hyperplasia: A stromal disease? Urology *16* (1980) 625–633.
[25] Ross, R., S. J. Klebanoff: Fine structural changes in uterine smooth muscle and fibroblasts in response to estrogen. J. Cell Bio. *32* (1967) 155–167.
[26] Ruoslahti, E., M. D. Pierschbacher: New perspectives in cell adhesion: RGD and integrins. Science *238* (1987) 491–497.
[27] Schwartz, S. M., G. R. Campbell, H. Campbell: Replication in smooth muscle cells in vascular disease. Circ. Res. *58* (1986) 427–444.
[28] Scott-Burden, T., F. R. Buhler: Regulation of smooth muscle proliferative phenotype by heparinoid-matrix interactions. TIPS *9* (1988) 94–98.
[29] Seifert, R. A., S. M. Schwartz, D. F. Bowen-Pope: Developmentally regulated production of platlet derived growth factor like molecules. Nature *311* (1984) 669–671.
[30] Smith, R., A. Nag, A. Syms et al.: Steroid regulation of receptor concentration and oncogene expression. J. Steroid Biochem. *24* (1986) 51–55.
[31] Storey, M., J. Sasse, S. C. Jacobs et al.: Prostatic growth factor; purification and structural relationship to basic fibroblast growth factor. Biochemistry *26* (1987) 3843–3849.
[32] Terranova, V. P., J. E. Liotta, G. R. Martin et al.: Modulation of the metastatic activity of melanoma cells by laminin and fibronectin. Science *226* (1984) 982–985.
[33] Thornton, M., R. Frederickson, L. Mata et al.: Collagen and the proliferation and differentiation of rat ventral prostate epithelial cells. Biol. of Repro. *33* (1985) 213–227.
[34] Turpeenniemi-Hujanen, T., U. P. Thorgeirsson, C. N. Rao et al.: Laminin increases the release of type IV collagenase from malignant cells. J. Biol. Chem. *261* (1986) 1883–1889.
[35] Wicha, M. S., L. A. Liotta, S. Garbisa et al.: Basement membrane collagen requirements for attachment and growth of mammary epithelium. Exp. Cell Res. *124* (1979) 181–190.

Steroid hormones, receptors and benign prostatic hyperplasia

J. C. Romijn

Introduction

The importance of steroid hormones, and in particular androgens, for the growth and maintenance of the (normal) human prostate as well as for the development of benign prostatic hyperplasia (BPH) is well recognized. The observation that BPH does not seem to develop in men castrated prior to puberty strongly indicates that testicular factors might be involved in the etiology of BPH. The general belief in a key role for androgens in the development of BPH has led numerous research groups to focus their studies on the various aspects of the presumed relationship between androgens and BPH. However, despite the overwhelming number of publications concerning steroid hormone levels, steroid receptors and steroid metabolism in BPH that appeared during the past decade, the precise role of androgens in the pathogenesis of BPH still remains largely unresolved. Instead, the different experimental approaches used have rather led to a large number of conflicting data. The purpose of this paper is to discuss some of these controversial issues.

Mechanism of androgen action

Before discussing the possible role of androgens in the pathogenesis of prostatic diseases it might be useful to consider the mechanism of action of androgens in the human prostate at first (fig. 1). Testosterone (T) is the major androgen in the circulation. In the blood part of the available hormone is reversibly bound to steroid binding proteins, such as sex hormone binding globulin (SHBG). As T is supposed to enter the cell in the unbound state, probably by passive diffusion, the concentration of T-binding proteins in the plasma could be one of the factors that influence the biological effects of androgens on the prostatic cell. Inside the cell T is converted to the biologically more active androgen dihydrotestosterone (DHT) by the enzyme 4-ketosteroid 5α-oxidoreductase (5α-reductase). There is strong evidence that 5α-reductase is localized predominantly in the nuclear

New Developments in Biosciences 5

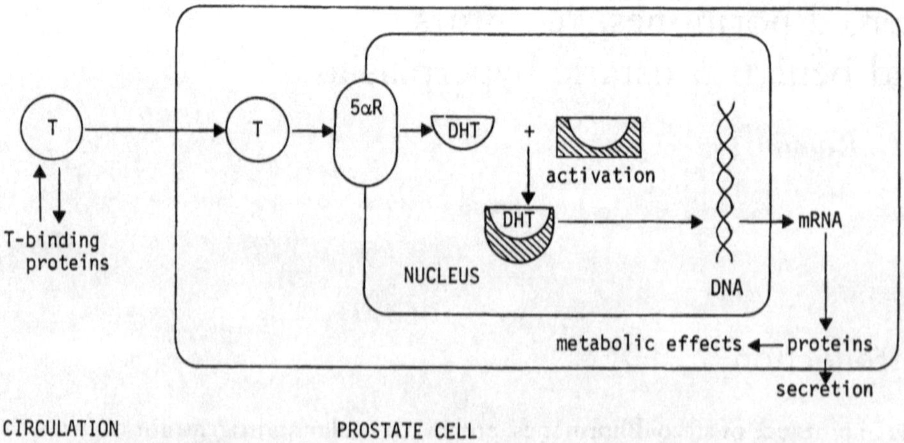

Fig. 1 Schematic representation of androgen action on a prostatic epithelial cell. Free testosterone (T) enters the cell where it is converted to dihydrotestosterone (DHT) by the enzyme 5α-reductase (5α-R). Androgen receptors are activated upon binding of DHT. The steroid-receptor-complex interacts with DNA and activates hormone-responsive genes. As a result specific mRNA and proteins are synthesized which may elicit hormone-induced responses in the prostatic cell.

membrane [14]. DHT-molecules might subsequently interact with high affinity receptors (AR) and thereby induce the conversion of the receptor molecule into an "activated" state in which the affinity for DNA is increased. Currently it is assumed – by analogy with e. g. estrogen receptors [32] – that androgen receptors are located exclusively in the cell nucleus, also in the unoccupied form (previously "free" receptors were thought to occur in the cytoplasm and to be translocated into the nucleus only after interaction with the hormone molecule). Binding of the hormone-receptor complex to the genome is then associated with activation of hormone-responsive genes. This ultimately results in the synthesis of specific RNA and proteins, that mediate specific (hormone-induced) metabolic effects and proliferative responses.

The possible involvement of steroid hormones in BPH pathogenesis

There are several levels at which the possible influence of steroid hormones on the physiology of the prostatic cell might take place (cf. fig. 1). If it is assumed that steroid-related effects play a critical role in the pathogenesis of BPH, comparison of a variety of endocrinological parameters in the normal and in the diseased state might lead to a better understanding of the etiology of the disease. The following parameters will be discussed in some more detail below: a) plasma levels of steroid hormones, b) tissue levels of steroid hormones, c) steroid metabolism and d) steroid receptor content.

Plasma levels of steroids in normal men and BPH patients

In an attempt to identify differences that could possibly lead to conclusions concerning the hormonal involvement in the etiology of BPH, several authors have investigated hormone blood levels in BPH patients and in normal men.

Table 1 Some reported changes of plasma steroid levels in BPH patients as compared to normal men

Compound	Reported change	References
testosterone	increased	[15]
	unchanged	[2, 5, 9, 13]
	decreased (a)	[24]
dihydrotestosterone	increased	[2, 5, 9, 13]
estrone	unchanged (b)	[5]
	decreased	[9]
estradiol	increased	[24]
	unchanged (b)	[2, 5, 13]
	decreased	[9, 15]
SHBG	increased	[24]
	unchanged	[2]

(a): "free" testosterone
(b): unconjugated estrogen only (estrogen glucuronides are decreased)

Some of the reported data are listed in table 1. It should be concluded that this approach has not been very successful, since it has yielded many inconsistent data (cf. table 1). Levels of testosterone, for instance, were found to be elevated by Hulka et al. [15], whereas many other investigators reported no significant differences in comparison to normal subjects [2, 5, 9, 13]; according to Ranniko and Adlercreutz [24] free T might even be decreased in the plasma of BPH patients. Similar discrepancies were found also for estrogens. With respect to DHT the opinion seems to be less varying and a (moderate) increase was generally noted.

In view of the conflicting data a general hypothesis explaining the role of steroid hormones in the pathogenesis of BPH can hardly be given. There are several reasons why the "comparative approach" might have failed. Firstly, many difficulties arise in obtaining reliable data for "normal" controls. The incidence of BPH is known to increase with advancing age. In addition, however, the levels of circulating hormones are age-dependent too. It is, therefore, pertinent to use age-matched normal controls in this type of studies. The lack of sufficient numbers of "young" BPH patients and the uncertainty about the (complete) absence of BPH in older "controls" has seriously hampered a reliable comparison between BPH and normal prostates. Secondly, the exact time of initiation of the pathological changes cannot be determined. As the measurements are performed once BPH has become clinically manifest (i. e. presumably several years after its initiation), comparison of the hormonal status might be of limited value with respect to the question of the hormonal involvement in BPH etiology.

Tissue levels of steroid hormones

To explore the possibility that increased androgen levels might be a causative factor in the development of BPH, several investigators have measured the endogenous concentrations of various steroid hormones (T as well as its metabolites) in BPH tissue and compared these to the levels measured in "normal" prostate tissue. Siiteri and Wilson [29] found no significant differences in the concentrations of T but noted a four-fold increase of DHT levels in the hyperplastic tissue as compared to the normal gland. Moreover, DHT levels were higher in the periurethral area (where BPH characteristically commences) than in the outer regions of the same gland [29]. The increased concentration of DHT in BPH tissues was, later on, confirmed by several other investigators [10, 12, 18, 20]. In parallel with the increase of DHT a depletion of androstanediol(s) [10, 12, 18, 20] and androsterone [12, 20] was sometimes reported to occur in the hyperplastic prostate.

More recently the reported findings with respect to the elevation of DHT in BPH tissues was questioned by Walsh and coworkers [31]. Their studies suggest that the DHT concentrations measured in normal tissues, frequently obtained after autopsy, are usually highly underestimated. Incubation of prostatic tissue at 37°C, even for short periods (less than 2 hours), reduced the levels of DHT considerably. Under the appropriate harvesting conditions the DHT content of normal prostate tissues was found to be as high as in the hyperplastic tissues [31]. This observation casts serious doubts on the earlier presumed role of DHT as a major causative factor in the pathogenesis of BPH.

Androgen metabolism in the human prostate

Based on the assumption that DHT accumulation might be involved in the development of BPH, numerous studies were initiated in order to find out how the presumed DHT elevation is accomplished. The metabolism of androgens in the human prostate is regulated by a complex system of enzymes. Testosterone, the major androgen entering the cell from the blood, can be converted into a variety of metabolites. One of the most important steps, the conversion of T to DHT, is catalyzed by the NADPH-dependent enzyme 5α-reductase in an irreversible reaction. DHT can be metabolized further by 3α- or 3β-hydroxysteroid dehydrogenase (3α/β-HSD) into the corresponding androstanediols; this step is known to be reversible. The (irreversible) conversion of 3β-androstanediol to triol compounds might play a role in the elimination of androgenic activity. The enzyme 17-hydroxysteroid dehydrogenase (17-HSD) reversibly catalyzes the interconversion between testosterone and androstenedione (as well as between DHT and androstanedione). It will be obvious that a change in *any* of these enzyme activities might cause a shift in the ultimate concentrations of several different metabolites.

In view of the reported accumulation of DHT, studies on androgen metabolism in BPH were focussed on the activities of 5α-reductase (DHT-formation) and 3α/β-HSD (DHT-removal). Most of these studies indicated an increased activity of 5α-reductase [6, 16, 18, 21] either or not accompanied by a decrease of the activities of 3α/β-HSD [6, 16] and/or 17-HSD [16, 21]. Such changes theoretically contribute to accumulation of DHT. Still, these data should be interpreted with caution as there are several fundamental problems that may complicate this type of studies. First of all, heterogeneity of the tissues presents a major problem. Prostatic tissue is built up with epithelium and stromal elements (also the stroma itself is composed of various cell types). Stromal-epithelial interactions play an important role in prostatic development and growth [8]. With the purpose to find a molecular basis for such an interaction, several investigators have developed methods for the separation of the different tissue compartments [7, 22] and employed these techniques to determine the biochemical characteristics (including enzyme activities) of the individual tissue fractions. The results obtained in our laboratory are summarized in table 2. The finding that the stroma has a much higher content of 5α-reductase than the epithelium is in accordance with the results from other published studies [7, 19, 33] with one exception [11]. The activity of 3-HSD was reported to be more evenly distributed over the tissue compartments [11, 19, 33]. With respect to 17-HSD our data disagree with those of Bartsch et al. [4] who measured a markedly higher activity in the epithelial compartment. It cannot be excluded that the results are influenced by the techniques used for the separation of the tissue fractions. With the procedure

Table 2 Activity of 5α-reductase, 3-hydroxysteroid dehydrogenase and 17-hydroxysteroid dehydrogenase in stroma and epithelium isolated from human BPH tissues

Enzyme	substrate/cofactor		products	enzymatic conversion (pmol/h. mg protein)		
				E	S	S/E
5α-reductase	T	NADPH	DHT + Adiol	5.0 ± 2.8	55 ± 34	12.9 ± 6.4
3α-HSD	DHT	NADPH	3α-Adiol	6.8 ± 2.4	4.2 ± 0.7	0.8 ± 0.4
3β-HSD	DHT	NADPH	3β-Adiol	2.9 ± 1.1	1.9 ± 0.3	0.7 ± 0.4
17-HSD	T	NAD^+	Adione + Aedione	8.0 ± 2.0	8.3 ± 3.3	1.0 ± 0.3

Epithelium (E) and stroma (S) were isolated from 8 to 12 different BPH tissues according to the procedure described by Oishi et al. [22]. Incubations were performed using radiolabeled steroids and cofactors as indicated; for determination of NADPH-dependent enzymes an NADPH generating system was used (0.5 mM NADP + G-6-P and G-6-PDH). The analysis of steroid metabolites was carried out using thinlayer chromatography as described by Schweikert et al. [27].

used in our laboratory [22] the epithelial fraction is of high purity but contains secretory epithelial cells (staining positively for acid phosphatase) only. Cultures of epithelial cells, in contrast, mainly contained the basal cell type (acid phosphatase negative) and had a 5α-reductase activity comparable to the level measured in cultured fibroblasts (unpublished results; cf. [27]).

Nevertheless, the observations made with separated tissue fractions suggest an uneven distribution of at least some of the enzymes. If this holds true, then the tissue composition (ratio epithelium/stroma) should influence the metabolic capacity of the tissue. However, the lack of correlation between 5α-reductase activity and epithelial content as observed in a large series of biopsy specimens [28] as well as in our own studies (fig. 2) seems to contradict this assumption. This might indicate that a second type of heterogeneity exists, resulting in regional variations that apparently overrule the differences between epithelium and stroma. Evidence for such regional differences has been presented in the literature [11]. Our own studies (fig. 2) showed that in 16 samples, obtained from the same gland, the activity varied from 3.5 to 98.7 pmol DHT formed/hr. mg protein. The pattern of activities was completely at random without apparent systematic differences between, for instance, periurethral and peripheral areas. These results implicate that sampling problems offer a major obstacle in studying the role of steroid metabolism in the pathophysiology of the human prostate.

Another point to be addressed concerns the technical aspects of the enzyme determinations. Necessarily the determinations are usually to be performed in artificial systems: either slices, minces and homogenates of prostatic tissues (or

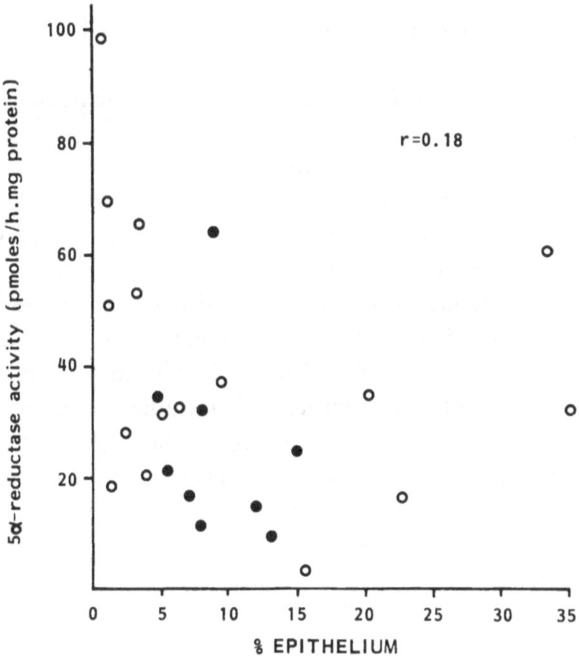

Fig. 2 Absence of correlation between 5α-reductase activity and the relative amount of epithelium in BPH tissue. The percentage of epithelium was measured morphometrically as the area occupied by epithelial cells relative to the total area of cells in frozen sections of the sample. Activity of 5α-rèductase was determined as described by Schweikert et al. [27]. Different symbols refer to (two) different prostates.

tissue fractions) or cultured cells (primary cell cultures or fibroblasts). In the case of homogenates the assays should preferably be carried out under optimized conditions (i. e. with relatively high substrate concentrations, addition of cofactors) and the results should be expressed in terms of V_{max} (maximal rate of conversion). The actual enzymatic conversion as it occurs in vivo, however, depends – apart from the amount of enzyme – also on the availability of substrate, the affinity constant (K_m), the availability of cofactors, and the presence of (endogenous) inhibitors. With respect to the affinity constant it should be noticed that recently evidence was presented that the (apparent) K_m-value of stromal 5α-reductase might be higher than that of the epithelial enzyme [25]. This implicates that the possibly higher concentration (V_{max}) in the stroma might be compensated by a lower efficacy of the enzyme. Unfortunately, most of the other factors (substrate and cofactor concentrations) are largely unknown. It is not unlikely that the exogenous supply of steroid hormones in the epithelium (being in less closer contact with the blood) is qualitatively and quantitatively different from that in the stroma.

A role for estrogens in the pathogenesis of BPH?

Referring to the increasing plasma levels of estrogens with advancing age and to the observed accumulation of estrogens in BPH tissue (especially in stromal nuclei [19]), it is attractive to speculate about a stimulatory role for estrogens in the development of BPH. Estrogens are produced in the male by aromatization of androstenedione (forming estrone) or testosterone (forming estradiol). Such a conversion, catalyzed by "aromatase" (a cytochrome P450-dependent enzyme complex) might take place in peripheral tissues (e. g. adipose or muscle tissue) or, perhaps, in the prostate itself. Some evidence for local estrogen production was obtained from experiments using cultured BPH fibroblasts [26] or whole tissue homogenates [17, 30]. In contrast, however, other studies (using assays of similar sensitivity) failed to show any aromatase activity in homogenates of BPH tissue [3] or tissue fractions (unpublished results). Therefore, local aromatization of androgens in the prostate remains a controversial issue. This does not necessarily exclude an important role for estrogens in the regulation of prostatic growth, however, although direct proof is still lacking.

Androgen receptors

In spite of considerable technical difficulties that have been encountered in androgen receptor (AR) assays, the presence of AR in BPH was demonstrated unambigously by a large number of investigators. As most of the receptor studies were focussed on the occurrence of AR in prostatic carcinomas and on its relationship with hormone sensitivity, relatively few data are available concerning AR in BPH. As part of a larger study, Van Aubel et al. [1] investigated the AR content of BPH and normal tissues by using a miniaturized AR assay that is applicable to small, biopsy-size samples. Their results indicated that somewhat higher AR levels were present in BPH as compared to essentially normal prostate tissue. Analysis of multiple biopsies, obtained from the same tumors, indicated that considerable variations may occur within these tissues: coefficients of variation ranging from 30% to 109% were found [1]. At least part of this heterogeneity should probably be ascribed to the tissue composition. The level of AR significantly correlated with the percentage of epithelium in the tissue [1]. Recently, autoradiographic studies confirmed that ARs are located predominantly, if not exclusively, in the epithelial nuclei of BPH tissue [23].

The role of AR in BPH still remains to be established. Undoubtedly the presence of AR is required for the expression of androgenic effects. Uncertain is, however, whether a correlation exists between the concentration of AR and the level of expression.

Conclusion

Several lines of evidence suggest that androgens, and possibly estrogens, are involved in the etiology of BPH. However, direct proof for steroid-induced pathogenesis of BPH *in the human* is still lacking. Moreover, the molecular mechanisms of a possible steroid hormone-mediated induction of BPH remain obscure, in spite of intensive research efforts. At the present time it cannot be excluded that steroid hormones only have a permissive role – rather than being a major causative factor – in the development of human BPH.

References

[1] Aubel, O. G. J. M. van, J. Bolt-de Vries, M. A. Blankenstein et al.: Nuclear androgen receptor content in biopsy specimens from histologically normal, hyperplastic, and cancerous human prostate tissue. The Prostate 6 (1985) 185 – 194.

[2] Bartsch, W., H. Becker, F. A. Pinkenburg et al.: Hormone blood levels and their interrelationships in normal men and men with benign prostatic hyperplasia (BPH). Acta Endocrinol. *90* (1979) 727 – 736.

[3] Bartsch, W., H. Klein, H. J. Sturenburg et al.: Metabolism of androgens in human benign prostatic hyperplasia: aromatase and its inhibition. J. Ster. Biochem. *27* (1987) 557 – 564.

[4] Bartsch, W., J. Greeve, K. D. Voigt: 17β-Hydroxysteroid dehydrogenase in the human prostate: properties and distribution between epithelium and stroma in benign hyperplastic tissue. J. Ster. Biochem. *28* (1987) 35 – 42.

[5] Brochu, M., A. Belanger: Comparative study of plasma steroid and steroid glucuronide levels in normal men and in men with benign prostatic hyperplasia. The Prostate *11* (1987) 33 – 40.

[6] Bruchovsky, N., G. Lieskovsky: Increased ratio of 5α-reductase: 3α(β)-hydroxysteroid dehydrogenase activities in the hyperplastic human prostate. J. Endocrinol. *80* (1979) 289 – 301.

[7] Cowan, R. A., B. Cook, S. K. Cowan et al.: Testosterone 5α-reductase and the accumulation of dihydrotestosterone in benign prostatic hyperplasia. J. Ster. Biochem. *11* (1979) 609 – 613.

[8] Cunha, G. R., L. W. K. Chung, J. M. Shannon et al.: Hormone-induced morphogenesis and growth: role of mesenchymal-epithelial interactions. Recent Prog. Horm. Res. *39* (1983) 559 – 598.

[9] Drafta, D., E. Proca, V. Zamfir et al.: Plasma steroids in benign prostatic hypertrophy and carcinoma of the prostate. J. Steroid Biochem. *17* (1982) 689 – 693.

[10] Geller, J., J. Albert, D. Lopez et al.: Comparison of androgen metabolites in benign prostatic hypertrophy (BPH) and normal prostate. J. Clin. Endocrinol. Metab. *43* (1976) 686 – 688.

[11] Habib, F. K., L. Beynon, G. D. Chisholm et al.: The distribution of 5α-reductase and 3α(β)-hydroxysteroid dehydrogenase activities in the hyperplastic human prostate gland. Steroids *41* (1983) 41 – 53.

[12] Hammond, G. L.: Endogenous steroid levels in the human prostate from birth to old age: a comparison of normal and diseased tissues. J. Endocrinol. *78* (1978) 7 – 19.

[13] Hammond, G. L., M. Kontturi, P. Vihko et al.: Serum steroids in normal males and patients with prostatic diseases. Clin. Endocrinol. *9* (1978) 113 – 121.

[14] Houston, B., G. D. Chisholm, F. K. Habib: Evidence that human prostatic 5α-reductase is located exclusively in the nucleus. FEBS Lett. *185* (1985) 231 – 235.

[15] Hulka, B. S., J. E. Hammond, G. DiFerdinando et al.: Serum hormone levels among patients with prostatic carcinoma or benign prostatic hyperplasia and clinic controls. The Prostate *11* (1987) 171 – 182.

[16] Isaacs, J. T., C. B. Brendler, P. C. Walsh: Changes in the metabolism of dihydrotestosterone in the hyperplastic human prostate. J. Clin. Endocrinol. Metab. *56* (1983) 139 – 146.

[17] Kaburagi, Y., M. B. Marino, R. Y. Kirdani et al.: The possibility of aromatization of androgen in the human prostate. J. Ster. Biochem. *26* (1987) 739 – 742.

[18] Krieg, M., W. Bartsch, W. Janssen et al.: A comparative study of binding, metabolism and endogenous levels of androgens in normal, hyperplastic and carcinomatous human prostate. J. Ster. Biochem. *11* (1979) 615 – 624.

[19] Krieg, M., W. Bartsch, M. Thomsen et al.: Androgens and estrogens: their interaction with stroma and epithelium of human benign prostatic hyperplasia and normal prostate. J. Ster. Biochem. *19* (1983) 155 – 161.

[20] Meikle, A. W., J. D. Stringham, D. C. Olsen: Subnormal tissue 3α-androstanediol and androsterone in prostatic hyperplasia. J. Clin. Endocrinol. Metab. *47* (1978) 909 – 913.

[21] Morfin, R. F., S. Di Stefano, J. P. Bercovici et al.: Comparison of testosterone, 5α-dihydrotestosterone and 5α-androstane-3β,17β-diol metabolisms in human normal and hyperplastic prostates. J. Ster. Biochem. *9* (1978) 245 – 252.

[22] Oishi, K., J. C. Romijn, F. H. Schröder: Cell separation and characterization of epithelial cells from benign prostatic hyperplasia. The Prostate 2 (1981) 281 – 289.

[23] Peters, C. A., E. R. Barrack: Androgen receptor localization in the human prostate: demonstration of heterogeneity using a new method of steroid receptor autoradiography. J. Ster. Biochem. *27* (1987) 533 – 541.

[24] Rannikko, S., H. Adlercreutz: Plasma estradiol, free testosterone, sex hormone binding globulin binding capacity, and prolactin in benign prostatic hyperplasia and prostatic cancer. The Prostate *4* (1983) 223 – 229.

[25] Rennie, P. S., N. Bruchovsky, M. G. McLoughlin et al.: Kinetic analysis of 5α-reductase isoenzymes in benign prostatic hyperplasia (BPH). J. Ster. Biochem. *19* (1983) 169 – 173.

[26] Schweikert, H. U.: Conversion of androstenedione to estrone in human fibroblasts cultured from prostate, genital and nongenital skin. Horm. Metab. Res. *11* (1979) 635 – 640.

[27] Schweikert, H. U., H. J. Hein, J. C. Romijn et al.: Testosterone metabolism of fibroblasts grown from prostatic carcinoma, benign prostatic hyperplasia and skin fibroblasts. J. Urol. *127* (1982) 361 – 367.

[28] Schweikert, H. U., P. Totzauer, H. P. Rohr et al.: Correlated biochemical and stereological studies on testosterone metabolism in the stromal and epithelial compartment of human benign prostatic hyperplasia. J. Urol. *134* (1985) 403 – 407.

[29] Siiteri, P. K., J. D. Wilson: Dihydrotestosterone in prostatic hypertrophy. I. The formation and content of dihydrotestosterone in the hypertrophic prostate of man. J. Clin. Invest. *49* (1970) 1737 – 1745.

[30] Stone, N. N., W. R. Fair, J. Fishman: Estrogen formation in human prostatic tissue from patients with and without benign prostatic hyperplasia. The Prostate 9 (1986) 311 – 318.

[31] Walsh, P. C., G. M. Hutchins, L. L. Ewing: Tissue content of dihydrotestosterone in human prostatic hyperplasia is not supranormal. J. Clin. Invest. *72* (1983) 1772 – 1777.

[32] Welshons, W. V., M. E. Lieberman, J. Gorski: Nuclear localization of unoccupied oestrogen receptors. Nature *307* (1984) 747 – 749.

[33] Wilkin, R. P., N. Bruchovsky, T. K. Shnitka et al.: Stromal 5α-reductase activity is elevated in benign prostatic hyperplasia. Acta Endocrinol. *94* (1980) 284 – 288.

Growth factors in benign prostatic hyperplasia

R. K. Lawson, M. T. Story, S. C. Jacobs, F. P. Begun

Purification and identification of the major growth factor in human BPH

We began work on prostate growth factor in 1978, when one of us discovered that tissue homogenates from prostate cancer were mitogenic for fetal rat calvaria [8]. This work was done to try to identify the factor that causes osteoblastic metastases in patients with prostate cancer. We then found that BPH and normal young adult prostate also contained the mitogen which we termed prostate growth factor (PrGF) [9]. This early work was criticized because others felt that we were dealing with a "nutrition factor" or a change in thymidine pool that accounted for the increased uptake of tritiated thymidine used as a marker of mitogenic effect on target cells. We did extensive work using total cell counts of labeled nuclei and labeled metaphase chromosomes in culture dishes. Dose response curves to thymidine were also generated in the culture system to determine the effect of the thymidine pool [11]. These studies proved that we were dealing with a true growth factor and not a nonspecific response in the culture system. The experiments showed that the addition of a very small amount of crude tissue homogenate to the test cells resulted in 100% of the cells undergoing mitoses within 24 hours.

A standard assay of growth factor activity was then developed to use as an endpoint in the efforts to isolate, purify, and identify the growth factor [15]. The assay utilizes second to seventh passage human foreskin fibroblast (HFF) as the target cell and tritiated thymidine uptake by serum down-shifted cells as the indicator of mitoses.

Studies were then conducted using a radiolabeled receptor assay for epidermal growth factor (EGF) and we were able to demonstrate that PrGF did not compete for EGF receptors and therefore EGF was not the major mitogen in our preparations [14]. We then embarked on a long and difficult search for a means to isolate and purify the growth factor. Table 1 shows the scheme that was eventually adopted which produced the greatest amount of purified material with the highest percent recovery from the crude tissue homogenates. Using these biochemical techniques, we were unable to purify the polypeptide to complete homogeneity and recoveries were exceedingly low – in the range of 1–5% [16]. We determined

New Developments in Biosciences 5

Table 1 Purification Scheme

1. Homogenization in high ionic strength buffer with protease inhibitors
2. Dichloromethane extraction (aqueous phase)
3. Ammonium sulfate precipitation, 30% saturation (supernatent)
4. Phenyl-sephrose (gradient elution with ethylene glycol)
5. Ultrafiltration
6. G-75, low ionic strength buffer
7. DEAE (elution with high ionic strength buffer)
8. Ultrafiltration
9. G-75, high ionic strength buffer
10. Con-A-Sephrose (unbound fraction)
11. Ultrafiltration
12. P-150, high ionic strength buffer
13. Ultrafiltration

that the growth factor is heat sensitive, protease sensitive, that biologic activity is destroyed by pH below 5.0, the molecular weight is 17.6 KD, and the isoelectric point is 10.2. We also found that treatment of the growth factor with 1.5 M salt resulted in dissociation of the growth factor from contaminating proteins and produced predominately the 17.6 KD molecular weight species [18]. The growth factor was found to stimulate a wide variety of cells to undergo mitosis.

The next major step was the finding that PrGF bound to heparin and belonged to a newly defined class of heparin binding growth factors. A new isolation and purification scheme using ammonium sulfate precipitation, heparin affinity chromatography and HPLC, produced highly pure growth factor with greatly improved recovery from BPH homogenates [18]. We obtained three antibodies from Joachim Sasse at Harvard Medical School, that were known to react with the amino-terminal, carboxyl-terminal and mid-sequence regions of basic fibroblast growth factor (bFGF). Our preparation reacted with all of these antibodies on western blot analysis which demonstrated that PrGF was very similar if not identical to bFGF [18]. We then collaborated with Fred Esch at The Salk Institute where highly purified growth factor from our laboratory was sequenced with the finding that the amino terminal sequence is identical to the predicted amino acid sequence from the cloned bFGF gene [17]. An interesting finding was the fact that the amino acid sequence of both human and bovine bFGF isolated in other laboratories was missing the first nine amino acids that had been predicted from the cloned bFGF DNA. The bFGF gene codes for 155 amino acids and the amino terminal methionine is cleaved in all isolated forms of the polypeptide [1]. A truncated 146 amino acid form that is biologically active, is isolated in acid conditions [7]. However, isolation at neutral pH in the presence of protiase inhibitors results in the 154 amino acid form that we have found in the human prostate.

We prepared synthetic peptides to various amino acid sequences from different regions of the bFGF molecule to use as antigens for antibody production. We now have a number of different antibodies that are directed to the whole molecule or to peptide sequences within or at the end of the molecule that are being used for assay purposes. Our present radioimmunoassay is capable of assaying bFGF in crude tissue homogenates from specimens as small as 30 mg. This means that one or two needle cores from the prostate can be studied for growth factor content.

We have also looked for growth factor activity in other human tissues and animal prostates. These studies have demonstrated a high concentration of bFGF in the human and bovine testes and human epididymis [19]. We have concluded from these studies that the previously described seminiferous growth factor is in fact, bFGF. Studies on the rat and dog prostate have also established the presence of bFGF. However, the rat has substantial additional growth factor activity which appears to be EGF [10].

Characteristics of FGF

The finding that a number of growth factors share the common property of binding to heparin and share a high degree of amino acid homology with bFGF (most are identical to or are truncated forms of bFGF) has focused attention on this group of polypeptides as playing a central role in growth control in many diverse organisms. The fact that the bFGF gene is highly conserved in many species including amphibian and avian strongly suggests this possibility [6, 7]. A partial list of growth factors similar or identical to bFGF is shown in table 2. The large number of factors reflects the fact that many investigators discovered growth factors in a number of different tissues and each factor was named for the tissue from which it was isolated, or for the responding cell type.

Table 2 Growth Factors Similar or Identical to bFGF

1. prostate growth factor	8. chondrosarcoma growth factor
2. osteoblastic factor	9. myogenic growth factor
3. endothelial growth factor	10. uterine growth factor
4. tumor angiogenesis factor	11. placenta growth factor
5. macrophage growth factor	12. cartilage growth factor
6. seminiferous growth factor	13. astroglial growth factor 2
7. hepatoma growth factor	

Basic fibroblast growth factor is found in most tissues that are derived from embryonic mesoderm or neuroectoderm [7]. Table 3 lists some of the tissues from which bFGF has been isolated. Melanoma, chondrosarcoma and hepatoma

Table 3 Tissue Sources of bFGF (mesodermal and neuroectodermal)

brain	prostate	tumors
pituitary	testis	melanoma
retina	epididymis	chondrosarcoma
corpus luteum	kidney	hepatoma
placenta		
thymus		
bone		
immune system		

Table 4 Cultured Cell Sources of bFGF

capillary endothelium	tumor cells in vitro
corneal endothelium	adrenal
lens epithelium	rhabdomyosarcoma
adrenal cortex	retinoblastoma
granulosa cells	
myoblasts	
osteoblasts	
photoreceptor cells	
pituitary follicular cells	
foreskin fibroblasts	

have also been found to contain large amounts of bFGF. Many cultured normal cells and tumor cells from human, bovine and rodent sources contain intracellular bFGF and deposit bFGF on the basement membrane in vivo and in vitro. Table 4 lists some of the cultured cells producing bFGF.

Basic fibroblast growth factor has also been found to be in high concentration in basement membrane substance and bone matrix [3]. In basement membrane the molecule is tightly bound to the glycosoaminoglycan (GAG) heparan sulfate. Basic fibroblast growth factor does not have a hydrophobic amino acid leader sequence needed for cellular secretion [20]. Therefore, heparan binding and cell secretion of GAG is thought to be the way the bFGF molecule is moved from its intracellular location to the basement membrane [20]. Recent work has shown that heparan sulfate is the GAG involved and that the property of basement membrane to stimulate cell growth can be destroyed by treating it with the enzyme heparitinase [13]. The receptors for FGF are located on the surface of the cell and intracellular bFGF is not able to activate these receptors. The mechanism whereby bFGF finds its way out of the cell to the basement membrane or intracellular fluid is key to its role as an autocrine or paracrine growth factor.

The biologic characteristics of bFGF include the following: it is a mitogen for cells derived from embryonic mesoderm and neuroectoderm, and induces cell migration, blood vessel growth, dermal wound closure, plasminogen activation, and activates oncogenes c-fos and c-myc [12]. The activation and modulation of these effects in vivo may be under endocrine or paracrine influence. Androgen, estrogen and cortical steroids have all been shown to modulate growth factor activity in culture and animal model systems. An even more important modulation of bFGF activity may be by way of transforming growth factor beta (TGF β) [2]. This growth factor is present in many tissues and has been shown to exert both strong inhibitory and stimulatory effects on bFGF activity in model systems depending on the cell type involved. For example, TGF β inhibits growth of endothelial cells and angiogenesis induced by bFGF, whereas it stimulates bFGF induced fibrostromal proliferation.

The role of bFGF in embryonic morphogenesis, tissue growth and regeneration, wound healing, angiogenesis and neuronal growth and differentiation has been extensively studied. This ubiquitous polypeptide appears to play a key role in these many diverse biologic processes. It is easy to speculate that a derangement in control mechanisms for the biologic functions of bFGF could underlie the pathophysiology of many disease processes. The following hypotheses are proposed which could link altered control of bFGF with stromal and glandular hyperplasia in the human prostate.

There are two general mechanisms whereby bFGF might effect prostate tissue proliferation. The first is release of growth factor by epithelial and/or stromal cells either by secretion of growth factor by an as yet unidentified mechanism or by release of growth factor from injured cells. Figure 1 shows a possible direct

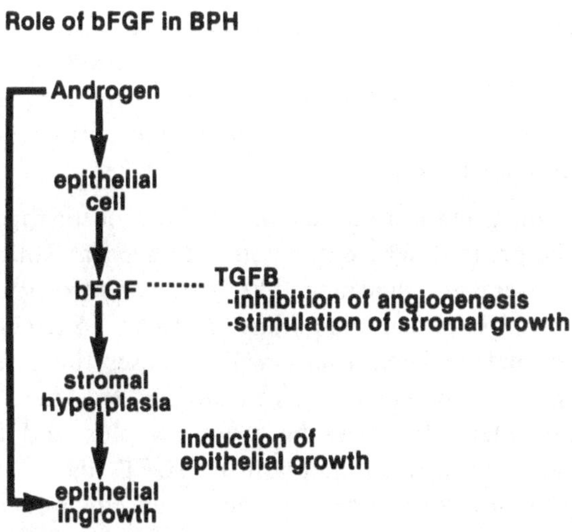

Fig. 1 Model showing possible direct effect of androgen on growth factor production and/or secretion with paracrine or autocrine stimulation of cell growth. TGF β may modulate bFGF activity.

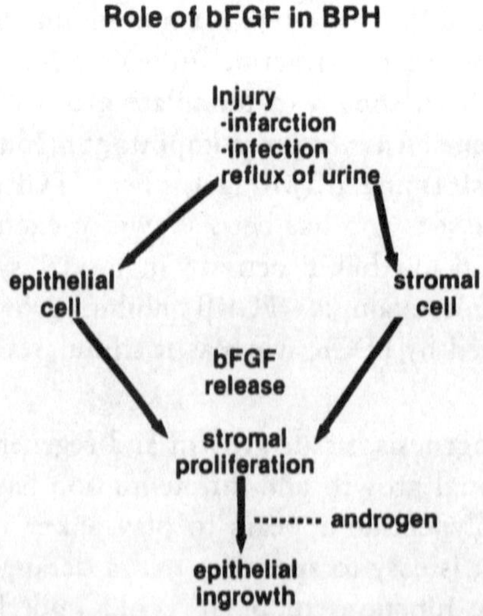

Fig. 2 Model showing possible effect of injury to periurethral tissue with release of bFGF from injured cells. Basic fibroblast growth factor then stimulates cell growth as an autocrine or paracrine factor.

effect of growth factor secretion on stromal hyperplasia caused by androgen stimulation. In this model TGF β modulates bFGF activity by stimulating stromal growth and inhibiting angiogenesis – both known effects of TGF β. The stimulated stromal cells may become a type of primitive mesenchyme which induces the ingrowth of glandular cells. This type of inductive effect of mesenchyme has been well established by Cunha [5]. A second model of direct effect of bFGF is shown in figure 2. Cellular injury might cause the release of growth factor into the extracellular space with paracrine or autocrine stimulation of adjacent cells and resulting stromal or glandular hyperplasia.

A second general hypothesis of growth factor activity is the concept that bFGF is produced by the cells in the prostate where it is bound to heparan sulfate and secreted as a component of basement membrane. The stromal and/or glandular proliferation then depends on cell/basement membrane interaction. Such an effect might be modulated by the enzyme heparitinase which causes the release of heparan/bFGF complexes from the basement membrane (fig. 3). Alternatively, the cell/basement membrane interaction may be more complex and involve autocrine or paracrine mechanisms with modulation by TGF β (fig. 4). Such a model postulates overall endocrine control through androgen effect on growth factor production and/or secretion.

Studies are currently being conducted to test these various hypotheses and include assay of growth factor concentration in various regions of the normal prostate

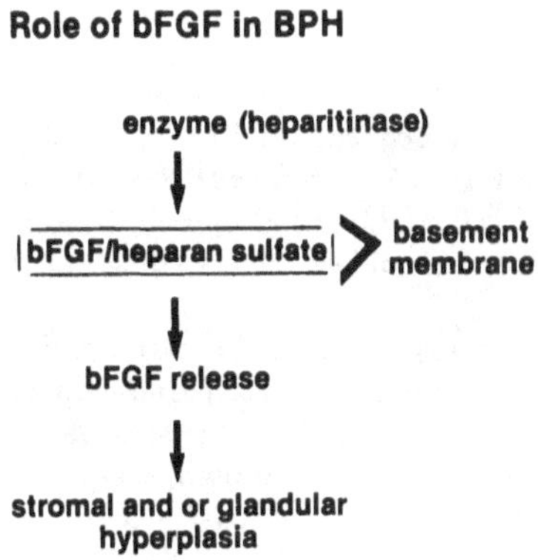

Fig. 3 Model suggesting possible role of bFGF release from basement membrane, by the enzyme heparitinase, in stromal or glandular hyperplasia.

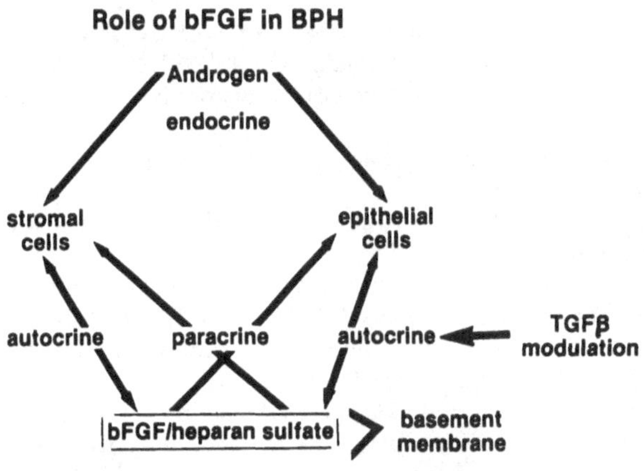

Fig. 4 Model showing possible endocrine, paracrine, and autocrine activity during cell/basement membrane interaction as cause of BPH.

and BPH, immunohistochemical localization of growth factor in various cell types in the prostate, and the study of effect of androgen and TGF β on bFGF production, secretion and biologic activity. The potentially important role of heparan/bFGF complexes in the basement membrane in modulation of growth factor activity is also under investigation.

In summary, we have isolated and purified the major growth factor present in human prostate tissue. This growth factor has been identified as bFGF by western blot analysis and amino acid sequence data. Several hypotheses have been presented which could account for a causal relationship between bFGF activity and the development of benign prostate hyperplasia.

References

[1] Abraham, J., A. Mergia, J. Whang et al.: Nucleotide sequence of a bovine clone encoding the angiogenic protein, basic fibroblast growth factor. Science *233* (1986) 545 – 548.

[2] Baird, A., T. Durkin: Inhibition of endothelial cell proliferation by type B transforming growth factor: interactions with acidic and basic fibroblast factors. Biochem. Biophys. Res. Commun. *138* (1986) 476.

[3] Baird, A., N. Ling: Fibroblast growth factors are present in the extracellular matrix produced by endothelial cells in vitro: implications for a role of heparinase-like enzymes in the neovascular response. Biochem. Biophys. Res. Commun. *142* (1987) 428 – 435.

[4] Baird, A., N. Ueno, F. Esch et al.: Distribution of fibroblast growth factors (FGFs) in tissues and structure-function studies with synthetic fragments of basic FGF. J. Cell. Phys. Suppl. *5* (1987) 101 – 106.

[5] Cunha, G., B. Lung: Glandular epithelial induction by embryonic mesenchyme in adult bladder epithelium of BALB/C mice. Invest. Urol. *17* (1980) 302 – 304.

[6] Gospodarowicz, D., A. Mescher: Fibroblast growth factor and vertebrate regeneration. In: V. Riccardi, J. Mulvihill (eds): Advances in neurology: neurofibromatosis, p. 149. Raven Press, New York 1981.

[7] Gospodarowicz, D., N. Ferrara, L. Schweigerer et al.: Structural characterization and biological functions of fibroblast growth factor. Endo. Rev. *8* (1987) 95 – 114.

[8] Jacobs, S., D. Pikna, R. Lawson: Prostatic osteoblastic factor. Inves. Urol. *17* (1979) 195 – 198.

[9] Jacobs, S., R. Lawson: Mitogenic factor in human prostate extracts. Urol. *16* (1980) 488 – 491.

[10] Jacobs, S., M. Story, J. Sasse et al.: Characterization of growth factors derived from the rat ventral prostate. J. Urol. (In press).

[11] Lawson, R., M. Story, S. Jacobs: A growth factor in extracts of human prostatic tissue. In: Prostatic cell: structure and function, pp. 325 – 336. Alan R. Liss, Inc., New York 1981.

[12] Muller, R., R. Bravo, J. Burkshardt et al.: Induction of c-fos gene and protein by growth factors precedes activation of c-myc. Nature *312* (1984) 716.

[13] Roberts, R., J. Gallagher, E. Spooncer et al.: Heparan sulphate bound growth factors: a mechanism for stromal cell mediated haemopoiesis. Nature *332* (1988) 376 – 378.

[14] Story, M., S. Jacobs, R. Lawson: Epidermal growth factor is not the major growth-promoting agent in extracts of prostatic tissue. J. Urol. *130* (1983) 175 – 179.

[15] Story, M., S. Jacobs, R. Lawson: Preliminary characterization and evaluation of techniques for the isolation of prostate-derived growth factor. In: New approaches to the study of benign prostatic hyperplasia, pp. 197 – 216. Alan R. Liss, Inc., New York 1984.

[16] Story, M., S. Jacobs, R. Lawson: Partial purification of a prostatic growth factor. J. Urol. *132* (1984) 1212 – 1215.

[17] Story, M., F. Esch, S. Shimasaki et al.: Amino-terminal sequence of a large form of basic fibroblast growth factor isolated from human benign prostatic hyperplastic tissue. Biochem. Biophys. Res. Comm. *142* (1987) 702 – 709.

[18] Story, M., J. Sasse, S. Jacobs et al.: Prostatic growth factor: purification and structural relationship to basic fibroblast growth factor. Biochem. *26* (1987) 3843 – 3849.

[19] Story, M., J. Sasse, D. Kakuska et al.: A growth factor in bovine and human testes that is structurally related to basic fibroblast growth factor. J. Urol. (In press).

[20] Thomas, K.: Fibroblast growth factors. FASEB J. *1* (1987) 434 – 440.

Transurethral prostatectomy – complications

K. Bandhauer

Introduction

The transurethral prostatectomy (TUR-P) is still the best therapy of BPH and in many urological clinics TUR is the most frequent operative procedure. TUR-P is also one of the fundamental operative methods which established the independence of urology as a speciality from general surgery. The increasing importance of geriatric problems in our western societies will further raise the need for this operation particularly as long as there is no acceptable and effective conservative therapy for BPH available.

Because TUR today is a routine procedure done on patients in older age and with more risk factors than usual intra- and postoperative complications should kept as low as possible. Therefore it seems necessary to review the complications of this operation continually and if necessary to improve the operative technique.

The importance of TUR-P as a urological routine operation has also to be taken into consideration for the training program of residents and we agree with the "Objectives for Residency Training" of the AUA after which each resident by the conclusion of his training must be able to resect 30 g in 60 minutes without injury or hemorrhage, describe vascular supply of adenoma, distinguish various tissues and discuss special urinary control mechanisms and their relation to resection.

To review our standard with the TUR-P we made a retrospective study to find out our results and complications and to look out for new ways in the future to further minimize the risks and complications. Therefore we examined the course of 3,500 patients who had TUR-P in our department between 1971 and 1986. The first group of patients was reviewed already 1976 and we compared this patient group with a second group between 1977 and 1986.

Although the fundamentals of the operative technique remained rather stable during these years we introduced minor but seemingly important variations in the intra- and postoperative proceeding.

New Developments in Biosciences 5

Operative technique

Instruments

In general Storz Resectoscope 24 F and only exceptionally when the BPH was uncommonly large (more than 100 g) the 27 F instrument was used. With the exception of 224 TUR-P where we used teflon coated sheats we employed metalsheats with high conductive lubricants. For irrigation aseptic (germ-free) water was applicated. The irrigation hight was between 50 – 70 cm.

Almost all cases were resected in peridural anesthesia.

Prophylaxis of TUR-P syndrom

At the beginning of the resection 100 ml Mannitol 20% and Furosemid 20 – 40 mg was administered intravenously to avoid hydremia and hyponatremia. The operation time was limited to 60 minutes and when venous sinuses were opened the TUR was interrupted.

The aim of the operation was a complete resection of the hyperplastic tissue up to the prostatic capsule. Exact hemostasis was practised and was the presumption for the use of small postoperative catheters (16 – 18 F) for 3 – 4 days. Until 1984 siliconized latex catheters, since 1985 only pure silicon catheters with a very smooth surface were used, providing good drainage of urethral secretion between urethral mucosa and catheter. Catheter irrigation was performed by a closed system.

Chemotherapy/antibiotics

Until 1974 prophylatic Furadantin was applicated during TUR-P and at least 5 days postoperatively in all cases without preoperative urinary infection, while infected patients were treated with antibiotics according to bacterial resistency. Between 1977 and 1986 no prophylaxis was used at all except in preoperative infected cases or patients with high risk factors like diabetes mellitus, chronic bronchitis etc. Because of three severe septic incidents with one death we changed this prophylactic strategy after 1986. Since 1986 we accomplished a one day chemotherapy prophylaxes limited to the day of operation with Trimethoprim-Sulfomethoxazol in preoperative non infected patients without risk factors. Otherwise the patient gets antibiotics according to bacterial resistency.

Results

The discussion of the results is based on the comparison between the two patient groups which were reviewed under comparable criterions.

Preoperative findings (table 1)

The most striking difference is the amount of patients with preoperative indwelling catheters. Permanent information and postgraduate courses for attending physicians and for laymen led to earlier diagnosis of BPH and to earlier admissions of patients with micturition problems to our department. Probably because of the same reason the percentage of bladder calculi was less in the second patient group.

Table 1 Preoperative findings

	1971 – 1976 n = 1014		1977 – 1986 n = 2486	
	Pat.	%	Pat.	%
catheter	414	40.8	628	25.3
renal insuff. crea < 1,3 mg %	104	10.3	176	7.1
urethral strict.	48	4.7	102	4.1
bladder tumour	26	2.6	75	3.0
bladder calculi	56	5.5	84	3.3

Intraoperative complications (table 2)

In spite of the usage of germ free-water for irrigation TUR-syndrom was a rare event, certainly due to the prophylactic application of Mannitol and Furosemid. The diminution of perforation and hemorrhage because of open venous sinuses was a consequence of better high frequency equipment with the automatically

Table 2 Intraoperative complications

	1971 – 1976 n = 1014		1977 – 1986 n = 2486	
	Pat.	%	Pat.	%
TUR-syndrom	3	0.3	9	0.4
perforation	8	0.8	13	0.5
open sinus	4	0.4	4	0.2

controlled TUR-system by Flachenecker and Fastenauer. The intraoperative complications were altogether rather low and a change of the resection technique is so far not necessary.

Severe postoperative complications (table 3)

No striking differences between the two groups appeared for severe postoperative complications except of the stress situation (stressulcera). A better preoperative instruction about the problems of TUR-P calmed down the emotion of patients and this kind of complication does not play a role any more. The three cases with postoperative sepsis were due to missing prophylactic antibiotics during the TUR-P with development of bacteremia. One patient died in septic shock. Since that time intraoperative chemotherapy prophylaxes with Trimethoprim-Sulfometaxozol is employed in all cases of TUR-P. In both groups no antithrombotic messures were used except in high risk cases like status embolicus, varicosity etc.

Table 3 Severe postop. complications

	1971 – 1976 n = 1014		1977 – 1986 n = 2486	
	Pat.	%	Pat.	%
stress-gastritis – " – ulcera	6	0.6	2	0.08
pulmonary embol.	6	0.6	7	0.3
apoplectic insult	5	0.5	6	0.25
myocardial infarction	4	0.4	5	0.2
pneumonia	4	0.4	1	0.04
thrombosis peripheral veins	3	0.3	9	0.35
agranulocytosis	1	0.1	–	–
ac. pyelonpehritis	1	0.1	2	0.08
mesenterial infarct.	1	0.1	–	–
shock kidney a. TUR syndrom	1	0.1	–	–
sepsis	–	–	3	0.1

Mortality (table 4)

Cardio-vascular incidences were the most frequent causes for postoperative mortality. This is understandable because of the age of these patients. All of them were over 75 years and were regarded as a high risk group. Altogether the mortality-rate in both groups is far below 1%, is therefore tolerable and justifies TUR-P as an excellent method even in patients with high age.

Table 4 Mortality

	1971 – 1976 n = 1014		1977 – 1986 n = 2486	
	Pat.	%	Pat.	%
myocardial infarction	2	0.2	3	0.1
apoplectic insult	2	0.2	4	0.2
mesenterial infarct.	1	0.1	–	–
agranulocytosis	1	0.1	–	–
pulmonary embol.	1	0.1	2	0.1
septicemia	–	–	1	0.05
	7	0.7	10	0.4

Moderate postoperative complications (table 5)

No difference exists in the frequency of bleeding during the first two postoperative days. All bleedings were controlled conservatively by irrigation or by evacuation of the bladder with coagulation of the bleeding vessel. Fibrinolysis never was the cause for postoperative bleeding. The difference in the frequency of severe urethritis was in contrast rather striking. Since using pure silicon catheters for postoperative urinary drainage this complication became a rare event just as postoperative epididymitis.

Table 5 Moderate postoperative complications

	1971 – 1976 n = 1014		1977 – 1986 n = 2486	
	Pat.	%	Pat.	%
fever < 38°C	51	5.0	142	5.7
bleeding	34	3.4	86	3.5
severe urethritis	11	1.1	6	0.2
epididymitis	4	0.4	3	0.1

Late complications (table 6)

Persistent urinary infection lasting more than three to four months after TUR-P can be caused either by pathological findings somewhere in the urinary tract (diverticula, nephrolithiasis, hydronephrosis etc.) or by prolonged "loge-infection". This infection is due to microbiosis of a residual hyperplastic tissue with deficient blood supply or to obstructive changes in the lower urinary tract like urethral strictures or bladder neck contractions. After the introduction of silicon

Table 6 Late complications

	1971 – 1976 n = 1014		1977 – 1986 n = 2486	
	Pat.	%	Pat.	%
Persistent infection	85	8.4	122	4.8
hematuria	20	2.0	52	2.1
epididymitis	14	1.4	12	0.5
temporary stressincontinence	10	1.0	28	1.1
total incontinence	1	0.1	2	0.1
bladder neck contracture	23	2.3	28	1.1
urethral stricture	14	1.4	21	1.0
meatal stenosis	11	1.1	15	0.6
incomplete emptying permanent catheter drainage	9	0.9	34	1.3

catheters some of these complications could be avoided and prolonged infections decreased significantly.

Late hemorrhage 8 – 10 days after TUR-P was in almost all cases connected with too early phyiscal exercise, as late epididymitis appeared in all cases after too early sexual activity.

Temporary stress incontinence – not to mix up with the frequent urge symptoms – appeared mostly in older patients with signs of cerebral sclerosis and disappeared in all cases during three to four months after the resection. Total incontinence, the worst disaster after TUR-P can be avoided by paying attention to the pericollicular tissue where the muscles of pelvic floor are closely connected to the muscles-sheats of the prostatic urethra.

Urethral strictures are not completely avoidable but they can be reduced by careful handling of the resectoscope and using lubricants with high conductivity for avoidance of thermic leasions of urethral mucosa (metal sheat – high conductive lubricants/teflon coated sheats – low conductive lubricants).

The almost constant percentage of urethral stricture in both groups in spite of better and smaller silicon catheters in the second patient group is explicable by temporary usage of teflon coated resectocopes with more late strictures compared to metal sheats. In the last years we are using only the metal sheats with high conductive lubricants and the frequency of urethral strictures were decreased significantly. The reduction of bladder neck contractures can be explained by the more careful resection technique for small fibrotic obstructive BPH with sparing trigone epithelium. Retrograde ejaculation should not be considered as a real complication. Loss of antegrade ejaculation appears in more than 80% after a TUR-P and the patient should be prepared for dry orgasm.

Discussion

TUR-P for BPH is an ambitious operation. The low mortality which should not exceed 1% and the low morbidity allow to employ this operation even for old patients. Exact handling of the resectoscope, basic knowledge of the problems of high currency, of the causes and symptoms of TUR-syndrom, elaborate and clean-resection technique, adequate catheter material and careful postoperative care are important assumptions for good results. Since introduction of forced diuresis during the operation TUR-syndrom due to hydremia is only a minor problem anymore and in cases of hyponatrenia concentrated sodium-chlorid infusions will solve the problem.

Although TUR or better, because TUR-P is a routine-operation, the technique should be taught carefully and each urologist should be aware that his professional and – last but not least – also his financial reputation belong on good results with TUR-P.

Summary

The intra- and postoperative course of two patient groups with transurethral prostatectomy (1014 patients 1971 – 1976/2486 patients 1977 – 1986) was reviewed and the results were compared.

Although the fundamentals of the operative technique differed only slightly in both groups. Some important variations were introduced (catheter material, antibiotica prophylaxis, high frequency equipment).

The mortality rate was low in both groups (0,7%, resp. 0,4%). Striking differences in the results of both groups were the diminution of perforation and intraoperative hemorrhage due to better high frequency equipment, of stresulcera and of post-operative urethritis due to better catheter material (silicon catheter).

Results of surgical management of BPH – TUR-P by cold punch technique

H. Bülow

Introduction

In 1962, Frohmüller, together with Thompson, reported for the first time in a German urological journal on transurethral prostatic resection using the Thompson resectoscope [13]. In January 1965, Frohmüller was named head of the Urology Section of the Surgical University Hospital in Würzburg. It was here that on March 27th 1965, he performed the first cold punch resection in Germany. Since then, this method has been established in several other Urologic departments throughout West Germany, and among others in our hospital.

Equipment and procedure

As opposed to the more widely known electroresectoscopes, the punch instrument employs a "cold" tubular knife for resection of tissue. Till about 1970, the punch resectoscope developed in 1935 by Thompson [14] at the Mayo Clinic was generally used. Then, in the early 1970's Frohmüller improved the instrument, working in collaboration with Richard Wolf Company [8].

A short summary of the fundamental differences between the cold punch resection and the electroresection follows [7]. Tissue is not excised by electrical means, but is resected with a "cold" tubular knife (fig. 1). This excision corresponds to the basic principles of surgical technique. High frequency current is required only for spot coagulation of spurting vessels. Resection of tissue can be directly viewed via a glass window, i. e. without the use of any magnifying optical system. The field of vision is somewhat smaller than in electroresection, however, but the contours of the tissue structures are more clearly defined. Very beneficial is the fact, that in case of profuse bleeding, the lumen of the instrument is not obstructed by an operating telescope or an electrotome, therefore vision can be kept substantially clearer by a strong flow of irrigating fluid. The cold punch resection uses a closed irrigation and suction drainage system, so that in order to empty the bladder, no part of the apparatus has to be removed during the whole

New Developments in Biosciences 5

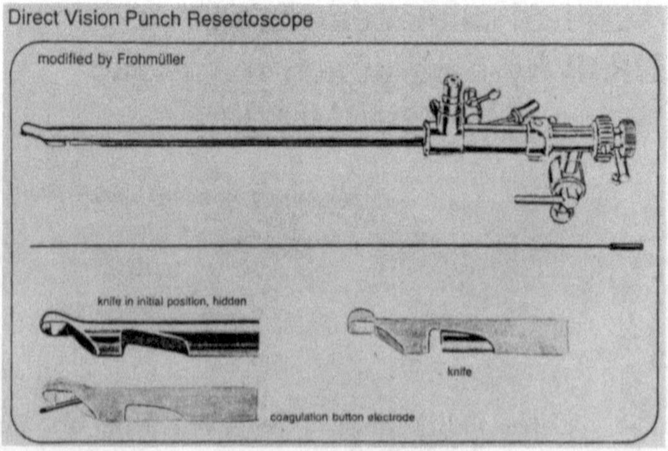

Fig. 1 Punch resectoscope, modified by H. Frohmüller

procedure. The construction of the cold punch resectoscope allows a tactile evaluation of the tissue. The experienced resectionist is capable of determining whether he is dealing with an adenoma, a carcinoma or with the so-called surgical capsule, based on the characteristic manner in which the tissue reacts to the resection procedure. The excised tissue is not altered by any thermic destruction which renders it very well suited for histological examination.

Cold punch resection, just as electroresection, is performed under a spinal or epidural anesthesia. In general, a nonhemolytic solution consisting of a sorbital-mannitol mixture is used as an irrigating fluid. Should a meatal stenosis or a urethral stricture be evident, or should it be apparent that the caliber of the resectoscope is too large for the urethral lumen, an internal urethrotomy with the Otis urethrotome is performed [9].

After completion of the resection and meticulous control of bleeding, the bladder is continuously irrigated with sterile physiological saline solution for about a 24-hour period via a 3-way hemostatic bag catheter designed by Frohmüller for this purpose [6]. The catheter is removed after 3 to 4 days.

Results

Between 1965 and 1985, over 4000 cold punch resections of the prostate gland were performed in the Department of Urology, University of Würzburg, Medical School. In 1978, the first 1490 cases were evaluated by Frohmüller and the author of this article [11]. In 1985, Frohmüller, Grups and Wirth published a report on 3030 cases [12]. An account of this report follows and is supplemented by cases from our own practical experience which were evaluated especially for this symposium. Since the establishment of our department of Schweinfurt, in 1981, we have performed 1235 resections of the prostate, 481 of them using the cold punch method, and these were performed only by the head of the department, the author of this article.

The average age of the Würzburg patients was 71.6 years, that of our own patients 70.3 years. In one third of the patients (33.6%), the operative risk was increased by a previous health problem. In 85% of the cases, resection was performed for BPH. On the average, 28.9 grams of tissue were resected, requiring 31.2 minutes. Hence, 0.93 grams of tissue were removed per minute. The largest adenoma weighed 155 grams and was resected in 62 minutes. Among our own patients, on the average 28.1 grams of tissue were removed. The average resection output was 1.5 grams per minute, clearly over that of the Würzburg clinic. This can be explained by the fact that among our patients, no training operations were involved.

The operative complications of the Würzburg cases are shown in table 1. None of these complications proved fatal. Table 2 shows the early postoperative complications. Complications resulting from the operation itself were vesical perforations, perforation of the rectum, postoperative bleeding and TUR syndrome. This constituted 2.5% of the Würzburg cases and can be explained by the fact that more than half of the operations were performed by residents in training. Among our own cases which were handled exclusively by an experienced resectionist, there were only 0.6% postoperative bleedings to be accounted for. Perforations or a TUR syndrome were not observed.

Tabelle 1 Intraoperative complications in 3030 transurethral cold punch resections of the prostate
(acc. to Frohmüller [12])

	Patients
Vesical perforation	7 (0.2 %)
Cardiac arrest	4 (0.1 %)
Acute cardiac insufficiency	4 (0.1 %)
Perforation of the rectum	2 (0.06%)

The surgical mortality rate after a cold punch resection totaled 1.4% for the entire period of 1965 to 1985 and only 0.65% for the period of 1975 to 1985. Among the cases in our clinic, there was a mortality rate of 0% until now.

Table 3 shows a survey of the most important late results in the Würzburg Department. We cannot report about late results in our clinic, since we generally do not see our patients again after their dismissal from the hospital.

Tabelle 2 Early complications following 3030 transurethral cold punch resections of the prostate (acc. to Frohmüller [12])

	Patients
Epididymitis	88 (2.9%)
Cardiovascular complications	70 (2.3%)
Postoperative bleeding requiring coagulation	42 (1.4%)
Pneumonia	39 (1.3%)
TUR syndrome	27 (0.9%)
Thrombosis	24 (0.8%)
others	15 (0.5%)
Mortality	41 (1.4%)

Tabelle 3 Late results after transurethral cold punch resection of the prostate (n = 581) (acc. to Frohmüller [12])

	Patients
Urethral stricture	21 (3.6%)
Incontinence	14 (2.4%)

According to the criteria, established by the Department of Urology at University of Würzburg, Medical School, a urethral stricture is diagnosed when the lumen of the urethra is narrower than 20 F [10]. Considering these criteria, the stricture rate of 3.6% can be considered as being low, since only half of these patients required treatment. As far as incontinence is concerned, the follow-up examination revealed that the risk of incontinence increases with the size of the adenoma and the length of time required for resection. There is no new evidence pertaining to the incidence and progression of perioperative urinary tract infections associated with a cold punch resection of the prostate. In an earlier report (1976) on the follow-up of patients who had undergone a TUR-P by cold punch technique, persistent urinary tract infections were observed in 24% of the cases 6 weeks after the operation [3]. Today this rate may be considerably less due to the intra- and postoperative employment of closed irrigation systems.

Discussion

The idea of a prostatic cold punch resection originates from the American urologist, Young, who, in 1909, introduced a punch instrument which, at that time, did not allow for a full view of the cutting procedure. In 1918, Braasch described a median bar excisor which made observation during resection possible for the first time. Not until 8 years later, in 1926, did Stern develop the first hot loop instrument [13]. The prostatic electroresection is, therefore, more recent than the cold punch resection. Nevertheless, the former has gained more popularity than the cold punch resection. What are the reasons for this? Are the results of the operation poorer after cold punch resection? Are the risks higher?

The same as for electroresection, there is no age limit for cold punch resection in patients with normal operative risk. Of the cases, treated in Würzburg, the oldest patient was 101 years old; of our own cases, 94 years old. Although one-third of all the patients had a previous health problem, the mortality was 1.4% and in recent years only 0.65%. This is probably in part due to the fact that the patients are virtually always operated under regional anesthesia. General anesthesia seems to be associated with an increased mortality rate [11]. However, this may only reflect a higher proportion of patients with a generally increased risk in the group of patients receiving general anesthesia.

The postoperative epididymitis rate after cold punch resection performed without a prophylactic vasectomy is lower than that after electroresection according to the majority of the published reports [2, 12]. A probable explanation for this is that during cold punch resection no thermic destruction of tissue occurs and the clean excision of tissue furthers a smoother healing process. Refrainment from electrical current may also contribute to the fact that postoperative contracture of the bladder neck is practically unknown as a consequence of cold punch resection. Likewise, dispensing with electrical cutting current offers considerable benefits for cardiac pacemaker patients [1, 12]. The voltage of the current, which is used for coagulation only, does not affect the fibrillation level of the heart. Whether refrainment from electrical current explains the low rate of postoperative urethral stricture after cold punch resection remains uncertain. Perhaps the reason for the development of urethral strictures has less to do with the thermic damage of the urethral mucosa and more with the existing disproportion in individual cases between the diameter of the lumen of the urethra and that of the resectoscope. In any case, a preliminary internal Otis urethrotomy, which was recommended by Emmett and coworkers in 1963 [5] and has been promoted by Frohmüller since, reduces the rate of strictures by 50% [10].

In recent years, Otis urethrotomy has been accepted by most electroresectionists, so that even large gauge electroresectoscope sheaths, for example those outfitted for continuous irrigation, can be used. In my opinion, continuous irrigation resectoscopes are not as time-saving as is the cold punch resectoscope, which is equipped with a closed suction attachment for irrigation fluid and pieces of tissue. Due to the rapid removal of relatively large pieces of tissue by the cold punch technique, TUR-P in combination with other operations can be performed during the same regional anesthesia. 2⁄3 of all patients with calculi subsequently had the prostate resected in the same session [4].

Thus cold punch resection seems to have slightly more advantages as compared to electroresection. Then why is it less popular? The fact, that cold punch resection requires extensive experience in direct vision cystoscopy, is certainly one important reason for its limited popularity, since most urologists are not trained in the use of direct vision endoscopic instruments.

During electroresection, vision may be considerably impaired by profuse bleeding, necessitating an interruption of the resection, compelling control of bleeding. Vision during a cold punch resection, however, almost always remains well maintained due to an intensive flow of irrigating fluid through the instrument. This is the reason for the experienced and speedy resectionist to find hemostasis an inconvenient interruption in the course of the operation and lets him postpone it till the conclusion of the operation. It requires a certain discipline, therefore, to perform a systematic control of bleeding at the close of each phase of the resection. The high flow of the irrigation makes it difficult for the novice, who is inexperienced in regulating the irrigation in order to recognize smaller sources of bleeding which can amount to a considerable volume.

Whereas the urologic surgeon is able to master the problem of hemostatis, this fact creates a handicap in regard to its propagation.

Trying to make the younger colleagues in training understand the necessity of dispensing with an optical device is rather difficult. A further handicap in the learning process is the fact that during a cold punch resection the field of vision and the exact site of the cutting procedure are not identical (see chapter of D. Utz). For the novice, this can result in substantial difficulties in orientation within the region of the operative process.

When the technical command of an instrument is difficult to learn, this is, of course, no valid reason against an operative procedure performed with such an instrument. It hinders, however, its propagation. Frohmüller, who masters the cold punch resection outstandingly, has in the past devised various technical improvements of the punch resectoscope and perhaps may find solutions to the previously mentioned problems. In the hands of the experienced, the cold punch resection is a fast and elegant operative method certainly equivalent to the electroresection.

References

[1] Ackermann, R., H. Frohmüller: Transurethrale Resektion bei Herzschrittmacherpatienten. Urologe *A 15* (1976) 185 – 187.

[2] Bülow, H., H. Frohmüller: Traumatisierung der prostatischen Harnröhre als Epididymitisursache nach transurethraler Prostata-Resektion. Act. Urol. 7 (1976) 77–81.
[3] Bülow, H., H. Frohmüller: Keimspektrum und Antibiogramm bei Harnwegsinfektionen nach transurethralen Prostata-Resektionen. Verh. Ber. Dtsch. Ges. Urol., 28. Tagg. S. 284–286. Springer, Berlin–Heidelberg 1977.
[4] Bülow, H., H. Frohmüller: Electrohydraulic lithotripsy with aspiration of the stone fragments under vision – 304 consecutive cases. J. Urol. *126* (1981) 454–456.
[5] Emmett, J. L., S. N. Rous, L. F. Greene et al.: Preliminary internal urethrotomy in 1036 cases to prevent urethral stricture following transurethral resection: Caliber of normal adult male urethra. J. Urol. *89* (1963) 829–835.
[6] Frohmüller, H.: Ein verbesserter 3-läufiger Tamponade-Katheter. Urologe *5* (1966) 144–146.
[7] Frohmüller, H.: Transurethrale Prostata-Resektion mit dem Stanz-Resektoskop: Operative Technik. Urologe *6* (1967) 166–171.
[8] Frohmüller, H.: An improved cold punch resectoscope. Endoscopy *8* (1976) 195–198.
[9] Frohmüller, H., H. Bülow: Use of the Otis urethrotome in the treatment of urethral strictures and congenital urethral stenoses. Eur. Urol. *1* (1975) 87–90.
[10] Frohmüller, H., H. Bülow: Zur Weite der männlichen Harnröhre, Konsequenzen für die transurethrale Prostata-Resektion. Urologe *A 15* (1976) 182–184.
[11] Frohmüller, H., H. Bülow: Die transurethrale Stanzresektion der Prostata (cold punch). Med. Klin. *73* (1978) 715–721.
[12] Frohmüller, H., J. Grups, M. Wirth: Die transurethrale Stanzresektion der Prostata (cold punch), Ergebnisse und Komplikationen. Urologe *A 24* (1985) 184–188.
[13] Frohmüller, H., G. J. Thompson: Transurethrale Prostata-Resektion mit dem Thompson-Resektoskop. Urologe *1* (1962) 171–174.
[14] Thompson, G. J.: A new direct vision resectoscope. Urol. Cutan. Rev. *39* (1935) 545–547.
[15] Utz, D. C.: Transurethral punch prostatectomy. In: J. F. Glenn (ed.): Urologic surgery, pp. 927–933. J. P. Lippincott, Philadelphia 1983.

Urodynamic implications of benign prostatic hyperplasia, parameters and suggestions for the set-up of prostatic studies

K. M.-E. Jensen, J. T. Andersen

Benign prostatic hypertrophy (BPH) is a process related to ageing and the most common cause of bladder outlet obstruction in male patients. Autopsy studies have documented histopathological changes with nodular hyperplasia in more than 70% of males aged 70 years or more [10, 16]. However, only 10–20% of elderly men develop symptoms and signs of obstructive BPH leading to prostatectomy [32]. This occurs when the growing prostate alters the conductivity of the prostatic urethra with subsequent changes in bladder and urethral function.

The urethra is not a rigid tube. Based on basic hydrodynamic concepts, Griffiths [18] demonstrated that the normal male urethra contains two constrictions. The proximal constriction near the junction of the prostatic and membranous urethra determines the flow rate in conjunction with the bladder pressure and the energy loss between the bladder and the constriction. The distal constriction near the external meatus controls the velocity of the urinary stream for the given flow rate. With prostatic infravesical obstruction the proximal constriction increases, and the urine stream through the prostatic urethra becomes turbulent due to irregularity of the urethral wall. This leads to increased loss of kinetic energy in the urinary stream. In prostatic obstruction, the loss of kinetic energy usually exceeds 90% [11]. The increased energy loss reduces the urinary flow rate – a consistent finding in studies of patients with prostatic bladder outlet obstruction [7]. The increase in bladder outlet resistance induced by obstructive BPH leads to elevation of intravesical pressure and detrusor pressure during micturition. However, both the turbulence in the urinary stream and the elasticity of the urethra imply, that simple calculations of so-called urethral resistance factors are not valid, since such calculations are based on hydrodynamic systems with laminar flow through non-elastic tubes.

The pathophysiological changes accompanying increased detrusor pressure generation also involve the contraction velocity on the detrusor muscle. Griffiths [20] found, that in proximal urethral obstruction, the "intrinsic speed" of the detrusor contraction was significantly reduced in spite of an elevated detrusor

New Developments in Biosciences 5

pressure. This has since been confirmed by Abrams and Griffiths [4] who found, that residual urine was not a sign of urethral obstruction, but a sign of abnormal detrusor function.

Besides hydrodynamic changes, BPH also leads to changes in detrusor reflex control in a large proportion of the patients [7]. The etiology and pathophysiology of obstructive detrusor reflex instability is still poorly understood, and further studies are necessary to elucidate this aspect of obstructive BPH.

In elderly healthy men without prostatism symptoms or signs of obstructive BPH, bladder and urethral function also undergo changes. These changes do to a certain extent overlap the changes seen in BPH, and this overlap represents one of the major problems in interventional studies of patients with obstructive BPH.

Urodynamic changes with age in healthy men

Flow

Only few studies have focussed on micturition in healthy male persons aged 50 years or more. Abrams [2] studied 86 healthy elderly males and found the maximum urinary flow rate to vary between 9 and 15 ml/sec. Similarly, Jørgensen et al. [29] studied urinary flow parameters in 93 asymptomatic healthy males in the "prostatic age" (median 64 years – range: 50 – 92 years). The variation in recorded maximum flow rates in 5-years age groups are shown in figure 1. The

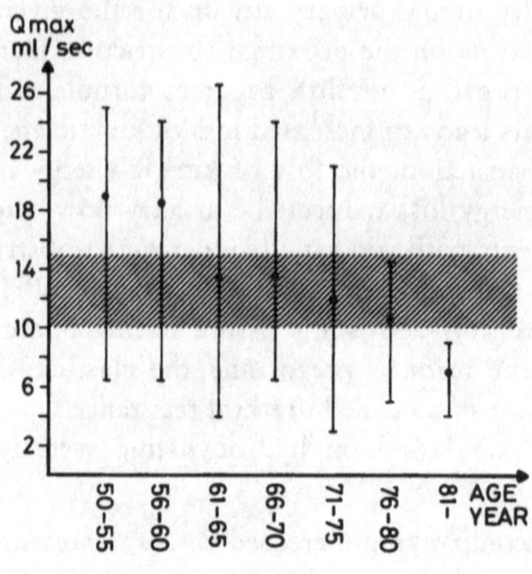

Fig. 1 Maximum flow rate (Qmax, ml/s) versus age (years) in 93 asymptomatic healthy males. Grey area: Qmax 10 – 15 ml/s. Median and range values are given. Reproduced with kind permission from the British Journal of Urology [29].

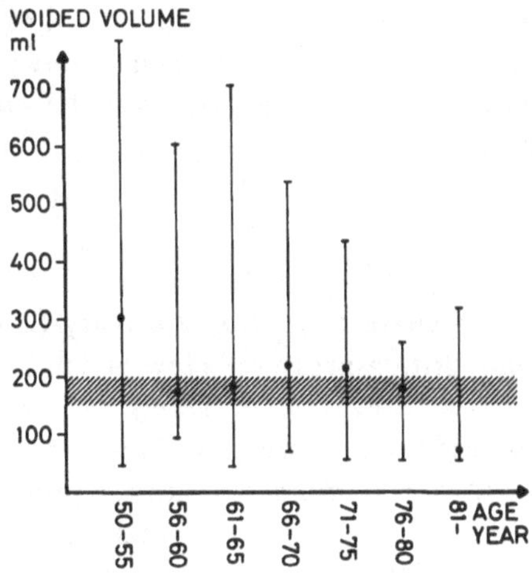

Fig. 2 Voided volume (ml) versus age (years). Grey area: voided volume 150 – 200 ml. Data from 93 asymptomatic healthy males. Median and range values are given. Reproduced with kind permission from the British Journal of Urology [29].

maximum flow rate is seen to decrease with advancing age from a median of 18.5 ml/sec at the age of 50 to 6.5 ml/sec at the age of 80. The hatched area in the figure depicts the so-called "grey area" in uroflowmetry. According to Abrams and Griffiths [4], flow rates exceeding 15 ml/sec generally indicate unobstructed micturition, whereas values less than 10 ml/sec indicate infravesical obstruction provided detrusor insufficiency is absent. In the "grey area" infravesical obstruction may be present or not. The corresponding voided volumes are shown in figure 2. It can be seen that the voided volume decreases with age. Nearly 50% of the persons studied voided less than 200 ml and 30% less than 150 ml. From figure 1 it appears that a large overlap exists in maximum flow rates recorded from healthy elderly males and from populations with BPH. The data imply that lower cut-off values than 10 ml/sec should be used in elderly males for discrimination between obstructed and unobstructed micturition.

Cystometry

Age alone may also change the control of the detrusor reflex. In a cystometric study of a series of healthy elderly males in the prostatic age group, Andersen et al. [5] found a prevalence of detrusor reflex instability of 53% (95% confidence limits 28 – 77%). A similar prevalence of detrusor instability was found in a population of patients with prostatism symptoms [7]. It is still unclear whether the age-related changes, i. e. deficient detrusor reflex control, are due to incipient infravesical obstruction, impaired spino-cerebral control of the detrusor reflex centers or a combination hereof. Although detrusor reflex instability in obstructive BPH disappears in approximately 2/3 of patients after prostatectomy [6], the results of preoperative cystometry is not in any way predictive for the symptomatic or urodynamic outcome of surgery.

Pressure-flow parameters

Micturition in the healthy younger male is characterized by a urinary flow rate exceeding 15 ml/sec and a maximum micturition pressure below 90 cm H_2O. In normal males aged 50 years or more, the flow rate decreases as previously mentioned. Only few studies have registered voiding pressures in healthy elderly men. Jacobsen and Andersen [21] found a maximum micturition pressure of mean 121 cm H_2O (range 95 – 150 cm H_2O) in 17 healthy elderly males undergoing pressure-flow study. These voiding pressures also clearly overlap voiding pressures registered in patient populations with BPH [7]. It thus seems that conventional parameters extracted from uroflowmetry, cystometry and pressure-flow studies are of poor discriminatory value in separating the voiding pattern in healthy elderly males from the voiding pattern in men with obstructive BPH.

Urodynamic changes in symptomatic BPH

The basic changes following proximal urethral obstruction are as mentioned decreasing urinary flow rate and increasing detrusor pressure, maybe resulting in incomplete bladder emptying und upper urinary tract deterioration. Recently Griffiths introduced the concepts of "Urethral Resistance Realtion" (URR) and "Bladder Output Relation" (BOR) [19]. The URR describes graphically the relation between pressure and flow rate during the entire micturition and thus defines the lowest resistance or the passive anatomical properties of the bladder outlet. Comparison of pressure-flow data with clinical data led to construction of a nomogram classifying patients as infravesically obstructed, equivocal or unobstructed [4]. The detrusor function was defined by means of the BOR, which is characterised by two parameters, namely the isometric detrusor pressure (pdet, iso) and the theoretically maximal flow rate, estimated as Qm, est = Q × pdet, iso/Δp. These variables are easily obtained from a stop-flow test during pressure-flow study. Patients with BPH typically have reduced bladder speed, i. e. Qm, est < 35 ml/sec.

These concepts have been further elaborated by Schäfer [38, 40] making use of computer technology. The inverse relationship between detrusor pressure and flow rate was stressed as well as the limited amount of mechanical energy available per voiding cycle. The pressure increase following obstruction was shown to be a passive adaptation due to the inverse pressure-flow relationship, rather than an active compensation. It was concluded, that the effect of increasing obstruction in BPH is a higher energy consumption per unit volume voided and that residual urine is a logical consequence of this myogenic limitation.

While the detrusor muscle provides the energy, the properties of the flow-controlling zone determine the actual distribution of energy between pressure and flow. This pressure-flow relation is described by the "Passive Urethral Resistance Relation" (PURR), and depends on 1) the urethral elasticity represented by the urethral opening pressure (p_{uo}) and 2) the effective cross-sectional area of the flow-controlling zone (A). These factors are linked together in the equation: $p = p_{uo} + \frac{1}{C} Q^2$, where C = a constant = $2 A^2$. In BPH, p_{uo} will typically be increased (normal value < 25 cm H_2O), referred to as compressive obstruction. Conversely urethral strictures will have a normal p_{uo}, but a decreased A and thence C, referred to as constrictive obstruction. This results in quite different graphic presentations [39, 40].

The functional state of the bladder outlet may also be delineated, using a modification of the PURR. From the equation above an optimal flow rate (Qopt) for all pressure values during the micturition may be calculated and then compared to the actually measured flow-values. These deviations ((Qopt − Q)/Q) are plotted as a function of time (Dynamic Urethral Resistance Relation (DURR)) and reflects the bladder outlet condition as influenced by neuromuscular factors (fig. 3).

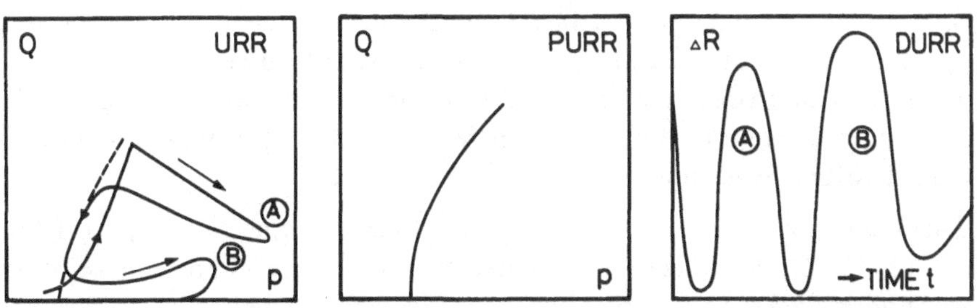

Fig. 3 *Left:* The urethral resistance relation (URR) demonstrating corresponding values of flow rate (Q) and detrusor pressure (P) during micturition. A = short time sphincter contraction. B = stop in voiding.
Middle: The passive urethral resistance relation (PURR) defining the minimum bladder outlet resistance as established by passive morphology.
Right: The dynamic urethral resistance relation (DURR) depicting active (muscular) changes in urethral resistance (Δ R) over time (t).
Modified after W. Schäfer [39].

In summary, detrusor properties dominate the voiding process, while the urethra has only a modulating influence on the pressure-flow relation. BPH causes increasing pressure and decreasing flow due to passive detrusor adaption. This in turn leads to higher energy expenditure per volume urine voided and eventually residual urine.

Suggestions for the set-up of prostatic studies

Prognostic factors for the symptomatic outcome of prostatic surgery

The search for prognostic factors in prostatism has been concentrated on data from conventional urodynamic investigations, i. e. uroflowmetry, pressure-flow study and cystometry.

Uroflowmetry

During the last two decades preoperative urodynamic testing has achieved an indisputable role in prostatism. Especially uroflowmetry has been widely used, although its prognostic efficacy has been uncertain. Several variables may be chosen, but the maximal flow rate is generally preferred [25, 31]. In open, nosographically orientated studies on prostatism uroflowmetry was judged valuable by several authors as to the preoperative workup [7, 9, 41, 42]. This view was supported by Abrams, who described an unsatisfactory low success rate of prostatectomy (72%) in a study with blinded uroflow [1], while the success rate improved to 88% following the inclusion of urodynamic assessment in the preoperative workup [3]. This result was explained by a high preoperative Qmax and predominantly irritative symptomatology in the failure group, i. e. they rather suffered from detrusor instability than infravesical obstruction. In general it was accepted, that patients with Qmax < 10 ml/sec were obstructed and would benefit from prostatic surgery, while patients with Qmax > 15 ml/sec were unobstructed. In the 10 – 15 ml/sec range the result was equivocal [7]. The voided volume was supposed to be at least 150 ml.

This reliance on urodynamic testing, however, was questioned by Bruskewitz et al. [12, 15, 23, 24]. Therefore a more comprehensive blinded prospective study was undertaken, comprising 139 consecutive patients being extensively examined pre- and 6 months postoperatively [25, 28]. The patients were classified according to the preoperative Qmax-values and in spite of differences in uroflow and pressure-flow variables preoperatively, almost no differences were found postoperatively. However, the high-flow group (preoperative Qmax ≧ 15 ml/sec) had a significantly lower subjective success rate (71%) than the rest of the patients (92%) ($p < 0.02$). This high-flow group was characterised by a higher incidence of persistent detrusor instability and a lower incidence of preoperative infravesical obstruction. Further analysis of the predictive value of Qmax confirmed 15 ml/sec as a rational cut-off value [25].

In conclusion, uroflowmetry is recommended in the work-up in prostatism, as patients with Qmax $\geqq$ 15 ml/sec do have a significantly poorer subjective outcome from prostatic surgery than patients with lower Qmax.

Pressure-flow study

The prognostic value of pressure-flow studies has been examined in only a few studies. As to obstruction Bruskewitz et al. found various pressure variables [23] and the minimum urethral resistance [12] of no significance, while Ball et al. [9] in a long-term study suggested preoperative detrusor insufficiency (low pdet, Qmax) as a predictor of postoperative failure. However, employing the nomogram of Abrams and Griffiths [4] in the above mentioned study of 139 patients, we found that obstructed patients fared considerably better symptomatologically (subjective success rate 93%) than unobstructed patients (success rate 78%) ($p < 0.02$). Although the two groups differed preoperatively in flow and pressure-flow variables, no differences in general were found postoperatively. Application of pressure-flow data on patients with preoperative Qmax $\geqq$ 15 ml/sec in fact defined an unobstructed group with a very modest success rate of 58%, which should probably not be offered prostatic surgery. Analysis of findings from the stop-flow test (bladder speed or Qm, est) revealed no prognostic value of the BOR [26]. This conclusion is in contrast to the findings of Millard in a retrospective study of few patients [36].

In conclusion, pressure-flow study analysed in terms of the URR has a significant prognostic value in prostatism, stratifying the patients in groups of high and low subjective success rates, while the BOR (using Qm, est) has not.

Cystometry

Several studies have suggested, that preoperative detrusor instability is associated with a low postoperative success rate, especially in case of normal uroflow studies [1, 14, 37]. As all studies comprised small patient groups and the cystometric data were not blinded, this conclusion does not appear well-founded. In contrast Dørflinger et al. [15] in a blinded study reached the opposite result. Our blinded study cited previously [27] also proved the preoperative demonstration of detrusor instability to be unimportant, both in terms of urodynamic variables and subjective success rate 6 months following surgery. Whether the patients were unobstructed or not did not affect the prognosis. Even grading of the instability was insignificant.

Conclusion: Preoperative demonstration of detrusor instability does not influence the postoperative outcome from prostatic surgery.

Routine urodynamic investigations in BPH

As shown previously by a variety of authors [25, 32, 35, 43] the success rate generally is high (85 – 90%) following prostatic surgery, even if urodynamic investigations are omitted, i. e. employing classic urologic selection criteria. Therefore careful symptom analysis and history, with regard to previous urinary retention, infection, current medication and neurologic or metabolic disease, are mandatory. However, as outlined above, stratification based on urodynamic investigations may further improve the prognosis and especially define groups of patients with a low postoperative success rate. The work-up consequently at least should include uroflowmetry and, if Qmax $\geqq$ 15 ml/sec, possibly also pressure-flow study. Cystometry may be indicated in patients with concomitant neurologic disease, but not in prostatism in general.

A follow-up program after prostatic surgery

Most complications following prostatic surgery will occur within 4 – 6 months (e. g. urethral stricture, residual prostatic obstruction, urinary infection) [35], where also uroflow variables and detrusor function will stabilise [8, 35, 37]. As 6 months appear too long an interval, especially if voiding problems are obvious, we recommend visits in the outpatient clinic 1 month (urine culture) and 3 months postoperatively (subjective evaluation, symptom analysis and uroflowmetry). If the voiding has not improved at the 3 months follow-up, and stricture and infection are excluded, a complete urodynamic investigation should be performed. Most often postoperative (persistent) detrusor instability will explain persistent symptoms, less frequently residual infravesical obstruction [27].

Suggestions for future research

"The risk patient"

A main problem in the preoperative evaluation of prostatism is to define the 10 – 15% of the patients, who will experience an unfavourable outcome of prostatic surgery. In our blinded study inclusion of uroflow and pressure-flow study in the workup actually did define groups with significantly lower success rates, but in fact the failure rate would only have been lowered from 11% to 8% [25, 27], which is not too impressive. Even an attempt to increase the prognostic information optimally by means of discriminant analysis of all our data was unsuccessful [28]. The main reasons were the relatively low failure rate and the high degree of overlap in urodynamic variables between the groups of successful and unsuccessful patients. Therefore conventional urodynamic testing hardly will solve the problem. Instead the value of sophisticated computer-assisted analysis of conventional studies as in the PURR-calculations, implying a more extensive utilization of the available data, warrants attention. Also bulbocavernosus reflex latency measurements [17] and evoked response studies [30] seem promising.

BPH and neurologic disease

So far the significance of concomitant neurologic lesions in patients with prostatism is uncertain. Most often cerebrovascular lesions and parkinsonism are encountered, causing detrusor hyperreflexia due to defects in the supraspinal control of the sacral micturition center. Generally these patients undergo comprehensive urodynamic testing preoperatively and still the postoperative outcome is less favourable than in patients with normal detrusor function [13, 34]. Therefore scrupulous clinical, neurological and urodynamic documentation of the pre- and postsurgical status, ideally as part of a protocol based on selection criteria as described for "pure" prostatism, might contribute to an unbiased evaluation and better prognosis of this common disease entity.

References

[1] Abrams, P. H.: Prostatism and prostatectomy: The value of urine flow rate measurement in the preoperative assessment for operation. J. Urol. *117* (1977) 70–71.

[2] Abrams, P. H.: The Investigation of Bladder Outflow Obstruction in the Male. Thesis. Bristol 1977.

[3] Abrams, P. H., D. J. Farrar, R. T. Turner-Warwick et al.: The results of prostatectomy: A symptomatic and urodynamic analysis of 152 patients. J. Urol. *121* (1979) 640–642.

[4] Abrams, P. H., D. J. Griffiths: The assessment of prostatic obstruction from urodynamic measurements and from residual urine. Br. J. Urol. *51* (1979) 129–134.

[5] Andersen, J. T., O. Jacobsen, J. Worm-Petersen et al.: Bladder function in healthy elderly males. Scand. J. Urol. Nephrol. *12* (1978) 123–127.

[6] Andersen, J. T.: Prostatism III. Detrusor Hyperreflexia and Residual Urine. Clinical and Urodynamic Aspects and the Influence of Surgery of the Prostate. Scand. J. Urol. Nephrol. *16* (1982) 25–30.

[7] Andersen, J. T.: Prostatism: Clinical, radiological, and urodynamic aspects. Neurourol. and Urodynam. *1* (1982) 241–293.

[8] Ball, A. J., P. J. B. Smith: The long-term effects of prostatectomy: A uroflowmetric analysis. J. Urol. *128* (1982) 538–540.

[9] Ball, A. J., P. J. B. Smith: Urodynamic factors in relation to outcome of prostatectomy. Urology *28* (1986) 256–258.

[10] Berry, S. J., D. S. Coffey, P. C. Walsh et al.: The development of human benign prostatic hyperplasia with age. J. Urol. *132* (1984) 474–479.

[11] Bottacini, M. R., D. M. Gleason, J. C. Byrne: Resistance measurements in the human urehtra. In: W. Lutzeyer, H. Melchior (eds): Urodynamics. Upper and lower urinary tract, pp. 301–316. Springer-Verlag, New York 1973.

[12] Bruskewitz, R., K. M.-E. Jensen, P. Iversen et al.: The relevance of minimum urethral resistance in prostatism. J. Urol. *129* (1983) 769–771.

[13] Cass, A. S.: Prostatectomy in vesical neurological disturbances. In: F. Hinman, Jr. (ed): Benign prostatic hypertrophy, pp. 776–781. Springer-Verlag, New York 1983.

[14] Cote, R. J., H. Burke, H. W. Schoenberg: Prediction of unusual postoperative results by urodynamic testing in benign prostatic hyperplasia. J. Urol. *125* (1981) 690–692.

[15] Dørflinger, T., P. C. Frimodt-Møller, R. C. Bruskewitz et al.: The significance of uninhibited detrusor contractions in prostatism. J. Urol. *133* (1985) 819–821.

[16] Franks, L. M.: Benign nodular hyperplasia of the prostate. Ann. R. Coll. Surg. *14* (1954) 92–106.

[17] Gerstenberg, T. C., P. Klarskov, T. Hald. In: Proceedings of the International Continence Society: Bulbocavernosus reflex measurement during cystometry predicts non-neurogenic and neurogenic detrusor overactivity, pp. 111–113. 1983.

[18] Griffiths, D. J.: Hydrodynamics of micturition I. Theory of steady flow through elastic-walled tubes. Med. Biol. Eng. *9* (1971) 581–588.

[19] Griffiths, D. J.: The mechanics of the urethra and of micturition. Br. J. Urol. *45* (1973) 497–507.

[20] Griffiths, D. J.: Urodynamics assessment of bladder function. Br. J. Urol. *49* (1977) 29–36.

[21] Griffiths, D. J.: Urodynamics. The mechanics and hydrodynamics of the lower urinary tract. Bristol: Adam Hilger Ltd. 1980.

[22] Jacobsen, O., J. T. Andersen: Voiding Cystourethrography with Simultaneous Pressure-Flow Measurements. Acta Radiol. *23* (1982) 605–610.

[23] Jensen, K. M.-E., R. C. Bruskewitz, P. Iversen et al.: Predictive value of voiding pressures in benign prostatic hyperplasia. Neurourol. Urodynam. *2* (1983) 117–125.

[24] Jensen, K. M.-E., R. C. Bruskewitz, P. Iversen et al.: Spontaneous uroflowmetry in prostatism. Urology *24* (1984) 403–409.

[25] Jensen, K. M.-E., J. B. Jørgensen, P. Mogensen: Urodynamics in prostatism I. Prognostic value of uroflowmetry. Scand. J. Urol. Nephrol. suppl. 114 (1988) 63–71.

[26] Jensen, K. M.-E., J. B. Jørgensen, P. Mogensen: Urodynamics in prostatism II. Prognostic value of pressure-flow study combined with stop-flow test. Scand. J. Urol. Nephrol. suppl. 114 (1988) 72–77.

[27] Jensen, K. M.-E., J. B. Jørgensen, P. Mogensen: Urodynamics in prostatism III. Prognostic value of medium-fill water cystometry. Scand. J. Urol. Nephrol. suppl. 114 (1988) 78–83.

[28] Jensen, K. M.-E., J. B. Jørgensen, P. Mogensen: Urodynamics in prostatism. IV. Search for prognostic patterns as evaluated by linear discriminant analysis. Scand. J. Urol. Nephrol. suppl. 114 (1988) 84–86.

[29] Jørgensen, J. B., K. M.-E. Jensen, N. E. Bille-Brahe et al.: Uroflowmetry in Asymptomatic Elderly Males. Br. J. Urol. *58* (1986) 390–395.

[30] Kimche, D., M. Saar, D. Lask: Evoked response studies in detrusor hyperreflexia due to infravesical obstruction in neurological patients. J. Urol. *133* (1985) 641–643.

[31] Layton, T. N., G. W. Drach: Selectivity of peak versus average male urinary flow rates. J. Urol. *125* (1981) 839–841.

[32] Lund, B.-L., E. Dingsør: Benign obstructive prostatic enlargement. A comparison between the results of treatment by transurethral electro-resection and the results of open surgery. Scand. J. Urol. Nephrol. *10* (1976) 33–38.

[33] Lytton, B., J. M. Emery, B. M. Harvard: The incidence of benign prostatic obstruction. J. Urol. *99* (1968) 639–645.

[34] McGuire, E. J.: Observations of a part-time urodynamicist. J. Urol. *129* (1983) 102.

[35] Meyhoff, H. H., J. Nordling: Long term results of transurethral and transvesical prostatectomy. A randomized study. Scand. J. Urol. Nephrol. *20* (1986) 27–33.

[36] Millard, R. J.: The clinical significance of bladder speed. Br. J. Urol. *56* (1984) 165–171.
[37] Price, D. A., P. D. Ramsden, D. Stobbart: The unstable bladder and prostatectomy. Br. J. Urol. *52* (1980) 529–531.
[38] Schäfer, W.: Detrusor as the energy source of micturition. In: F. Hinman, Jr. (ed): Benign prostatic hypertrophy, pp. 450–469. Springer-Verlag, New York–Heidelberg–Berlin 1983.
[39] Schäfer, W.: The contribution of the bladder outlet to the relation between pressure and flow rate during micturition. In: F. Hinman, Jr. (ed): Benign prostatic hypertrophy, pp. 470–496. Springer-Verlag, New York–Heidelberg–Berlin 1983.
[40] Schäfer, W.: Urethral resistance? Urodynamic concepts of physiological and pathological bladder outlet function during voiding. Neurourol. Urodynam. *4* (1985) 161–201.
[41] Scott, F. B., D. Cardus, E. M. Quesada et al.: Uroflowmetry before and after prostatectomy. Southern Med. J. *60* (1967) 948–952.
[42] Shoukry, I., J. G. Susset, M. M. Elhilali et al.: Role of uroflowmetry in the assessment of lower urinary tract obstruction in adult males. Br. J. Urol. *47* (1975) 559–566.
[43] Singh, M., G. C. Tresidder, J. P. Blandy: The evaluation of transurethral resection for benign enlargement of the prostate. Br. J. Urol. *45* (1973) 93–102.

Conservative nonhormonal treatment of patients with benign prostatic hyperplasia

K. Dreikorn, R. Richter

Introduction

Although considerable progress has been achieved in the understanding of the complicated interactive factors which are involved in the development of benign prostatic hyperplasia (BPH), hormonal manipulations have so far not succeeded in replacement of operative management in most of these patients [26, 81]. Therefore and especially because of the considerable side effects involved in the use of endocrine therapy many investigators have focussed on trials with non-hormonal agents. In the following, a critical review about the current status of medical therapy for BPH is given. As there is a lot of controversy in the literature it is difficult to distinguish "facts from fictions".

For each group of agents discussed the currently suggested theoretical aspects are outlined, the most important experimental and clinical data are presented and critically evaluated. The benefit of treatment with regard to the degree of subjective and objective improvement has to be measured against the severity and rate of side effects.

The obstructive signs of BPH are primarily a slow start of micturition, a poor or intermittent stream and a terminal dribble [79].

However, up to 80% of men with symptomatic BPH have secondary symptoms of frequency, urgency and nocturia, which, according to cystometric examinations by Andersen [6, 7], Abrams [1, 3] and Turner-Warwick [79], are due to associated detrusor hyperactivity ("instable bladder").

The mechanism, how obstruction should cause detrusor instability and why it disappears in only 70% of patients after prostatic surgery is unknown.

Calcium antagonists

Calcium antagonists, by their effect on vesicourethral smooth muscle can be expected to have an effect on bladder instability [39], Bödeker [11] described a beneficial effect of 10 mg nifedipine in two out of 5 (!) patients with BPH.

New Developments in Biosciences 5

However, as calcium channel blockers (nifedipine, verapamil, diltiazem) are potent vasodilatators they should be reserved for the treatment of cardiovascular diseases. From our experience in the treatment of detrusor hyperreflexia (neurogenic cause of detrusor hyperactivity) we know that there are more efficient drugs available today (trospium chloride, oxybutyine chloride, propiverin, emepromium bromide). The use of these drugs in vesicourethral obstruction, like BPH, however is not advisable, because they may lead to complete urinary retention.

α-Adrenergic blockers

In vitro studies, performed by Caine [21], have shown that α-adrenergic receptors are present in the human prostate, its capsule and in the bladder neck. Moreover, as urinary retention in patients with BPH can be observed after treatment with sympathomimetic drugs and often can be relieved by α-adrenergic blockers, it is suggested that α-adrenergic stimulation might be an important contribution factor in BPH – related obstructive signs and symptoms [12, 17, 18, 19, 20, 21].

Thus Caine developed the concept of an α-adrenergically mediated, so called dynamic component of variable degree in addition to the mechanical component of the anatomically present bulk of the hyperplastic prostate [17]. According to intraurethral pressure monitoring Furuya [40] suggested that 40% of the total urethral pressure in patients with BPH is due to α-adrenergic tone. Of the various α-blockers available, (phenoxybenzamine, phentolamine, prazosin, nicergoline, thymoxamine) phenoxybenzamine has been most thoroughly investigated.

Many studies, including double-blind placebo-controlled trials, have shown to reduce BPH-associated symptoms in about 70% of cases [17, 18, 20, 21, 41].

Moreover, improvement of voiding pressure parameters, increase of bladder capacity and reduction of urethral closure pressure was noted, unstable detrusor contractions were inhibited. However, Brooks [15] in a controlled study and Ferrie [36] in a double blind study found phenoxybenzamine in low dosage (10 mg/day) ineffective.

Side effects have been noted in 30–46% of the patients (hypotension, reflex tachycardia, weakness, dizziness, stuffiness of nose, retrograde ejaculation).

A major problem of phenoxybenzamine is its possible carcinogenicity, demonstrated in mice and rats, although no clinical evidence has been reported so far.

Nevertheless the indication of phenoxybenzamine in the USA and FRG is recommended to be restricted to its use in neurogenic bladder dysfunction and pheochromocytoma.

Prazosin, which is used for the treatment of hypertension seems to be a good alternative to phenoxybenzamine, because of its selective action on the α-1-receptors and fewer side effects [17, 45, 69]. Ronchi [58] in a double-blind crossover study found nicergoline to improve irritative symptoms significantly more than placebo. In 10 patients peak and mean flow rates increased by 50% and 77% respectively. No side effects were observed. In conclusion, the "two component concept" of Caine in patients with BPH seems reasonable and α-adrenergic blockage makes sense. The ideal drug with good effect and absence of side effects to replace phenoxybenzamine has yet to be found.

Cholesterol-lowering agents

It is well recognized that the prostatic secretion and the gland itself contain cholesterol [42, 69, 70]. Swyer [76] and Goldstein [42] found the cholesterol content of BPH-tissue to be twofold higher compared to non hyperplastic glands. The assumption that an alteration of cholesterol production and metabolism might be an etiological factor in the development of BPH motivated some investigators to evaluate the effect of cholesterol-lowering drugs on prostatic growth [43, 61].

Experimental studies in the dog showed that some polyene macrolide antifungal antibiotics (candicidin, amphotericin B, nystatin) significantly decrease serum and prostatic cholesterol concentration as well as prostate volume with none or only slight alteration of histology.

As these drugs are not absorbed from the gastrointestinal tract it may be concluded that polyene macrolides bind cholesterol and inhibit its absorption in the enterohepatic circulation. The exact mechanism of action of these drugs on prostatic growth is obscure.

Possibly the cholesterol metabolites 5α- and 6α-epoxy cholesterol which are known to be mutagenic and cytotoxic play a role in the formation of BPH and even in prostatic cancer as these metabolites are found significantly increased in both diseases [56, 61].

Of the various drugs tested experimentally, candicidin showed to be most effective, reducing the prostate volumes and weights by 33–67%, when given to dogs in doses of 5–30 mg daily. Other polyene macrolides like amphotericin B and nystatin showed less pronounced effects [61].

Human studies with oral candicidin reduced subjective symptoms in 89% of patients with BPH, and lead to a decrease of residual urine in 86%, an increase of flow rate in 89%, compared to 18%, 17% and 18% respectively, of the placebo-treated patients [49, 54, 73]. However, a critical review of Keshin's [49] and Orkin's [54] studies reveals that the controls were not adequate and that the objective parameters were not clearly defined to substantiate the conclusions. Scott [68] reported candicidin not to be benificial but associated with high rates of side effects like nausea and vomiting. Abrams in 1977, in a prospective double blind trial over 6 months, did not find candicidin superior to placebo [2]. The reported incidence of 60% in the improvement of micturition in the controls stresses the wellknown placebo effect in the conservative management of BPH patients.

Other agents with lipid- and cholesterol-lowering effect (bile acid sequestering resins like cholestyramine and colestipol, metabolic inhibitors like clofibrate and simfibrate) have not been investigated in the clinical management of BPH. Experimental data are inconclusive [61]. Side effects may be unacceptable.

In summary, especially because of the unknown mechanism how cholesterol-lowering agents should influence human prostatic growth, the divergent findings in clinical studies and the side effects reported by some authors, the benefit of these drugs remains controversial.

Phytotherapeutic drugs

Extracts from plants have been tried since ancient times for the treatment of BPH-associated symptoms, as can be read in the old Egyptian Papyrus, dated of the 15th century BC [33, 34].

Phytotherapeutic drugs are still very popular in West Germany. According to a drug prescription report the total sales of the most popular 16 phytotherapeutic drugs used in 1986 amounted to 131 millions Deutsch Marks [65].

The plants used most frequently for extracts are hypoxis rooperi, the leaves and roots of urtica dioica and urens, sabal serrulatum, pumpkin seeds (curcurbita pepo), pygeum africanum, populus tremula, echinacea purpura and secale cereale. Table 1 shows a selection of drugs available and their origin. The suggested effects of phytotherapeutic drugs are explained by most manufacturers by their content of phytosterols of which sitosterols are supposed to be the most important agents. Chemically the sitosterols resemble cholesterol. The mechanism of action of sitosterols is unknown. According to some investigators sitosterols interfere with prostaglandin synthesis and its metabolism in the prostate, reducing BPH-associated symptoms by an experimentally demonstrated antiinflammatory effect [9, 44, 51, 56, 57, 75]. Because phytosterols are poorly absorbed, other authors explain their effect by their cholesterol-lowering action through binding of cholesterol in the gastrointestinal tract [83]. However, about 10 g of sitosterols

Table 1 a Origin of "phytotherapeutic drugs" used in the management of patients with BPH

1. Hypoxis rooperi	5. Pygeum africanum
2. Herba and/or Radix urticae	6. Populus tremula
3. Sabal serrulatum	7. Echinacea purpura
4. Cucurbita pepo	8. Secale cereale (Extr. Pollin. sicc.)

Table 1 b Selection of phytotherapeutic drugs® available in the FRG

Azuprostat (7, x)	Prostasal (x)
Bazoton (2)	Prostaselect (3)
Cysto Fink (4)	Prostatin (2, 4)
Cernilton (8)	Prostavigol (3)
Eviprostat (6)	Protitis Drg. (3)
Harzol (1)	Remigeron (3)
Hewesabal (2, 3, 4)	Salus Kürbis T. comp. (2, 3, 4, 7)
Nomon (4, 7)	Sito – Lande (x)
Prostaforton (7, x)	Sitosterin Delalande (x)
Prostagutt (2, 3, 6)	Sitosterin Prostata K (x)
Prostaherb N (2)	Spasmo Urgenin (3, 7)
Prosta Fink (3, 4, 7)	Triastonal (x)
Prostamed (4, 6)	Urgenin (3, 7)
Prostagalen (2, 3)	Urtica Plus (2)

Origin given in ( ), see table 1 a.
x: β-sitosterol, origin not stated by manufacturer

daily are necessary to lower the plasma cholesterol level by 10–20%. Most of the phytotherapeutic drugs only contain about 10 mg per tablet. Moreover, 175–200 mg of sitosterols are consumed daily by the intake of ordinary food [46].

The action of extracts from radix urticae has been explained by the reduction of the sex hormone binding globuline (SHBG) [64, 74, 75, 77, 80]. However, the age associated increase of SHBG is observed in men with and without symptomatic BPH, making the significance of SHBG in BPH difficult to explain [49]. A direct effect of the extracts on prostatic tissue is more than questionable [10, 84].

A huge number of publications exists, describing the effects of phytodrugs in the treatment of BPH in stage I and II (table 2 and 3). Subjective improvement is rated in 60–80%. However, similar rates were recorded in controls.

Some authors and manufacturers state, that the 10% content of β-sitosterol-D-glucoside in their preparations might be important [55]. However, in a double blind trial of Kadow [48] 0,3 mg/day of the drug over 6 months has not shown to be superior to placebo, when urodynamic criteria were evaluated.

Table 2 Selection of publications concerning the clinical effect of phytotherapeutic drugs in patients with BPH

kind of study	no. pts.	drug tested	"subjective improvement"	objective improvement	author	year	(ref.)
open	2000	β-sitosterol	90%	↓ res. urine 70%	Ebbinghaus	1974	[31]
double blind	50	β-sitosterol	?	pfr ↑, res. urine ↓	Ebbinghaus	1977	[32]
open	20	β-sitosterol	70%	–	Tunn	1978	[78]
open	53	β-sitosterol	98%	pfr ↑ mfr ↑	Albrecht	1981	[4]
open	20	β-sitosterol	?	pfr ↑ mfr ↑	Klingeberg	1981	[50]
open	449	β-sitosterol	83%	↓ res. urine	Rummani	1981	[59]
open	105	ERU	75%	pfr ↑ res. urine ↓	Djulepa	1982	[28]
multicenter	114	β-sitosterol	100%	res. urine ↓ pfr ↑	Dressler	1983	[30]
multicenter	5307	sitosterol	89%	pfr ↑, res. urine ↓	Schindler	1983	[63]
multicenter	5492	ERU	61–83%	?	Tosch	1983	[77]
multicenter	4051	ERU	68%	–	Stahl	1984	[74]
multicenter	5054	β-sitosterol	86%	↓ res. urine 79,8%	Brühl	1985	[16]
double blind	147	Sem. Cucurb.	48% (29%)	? ?	Schilcher	1985	[62]
double blind	50	ERU	= placebo	pfr ↑ mv ↑	Vontobel	1985	[80]
multicenter	14574	β-sitosterol	81%	? ?	Schneider	1986	[66]
multicenter	149	ERHU	91,7%	pfr ↑ res. urine ↓	Brandstädter	1987	[14]
double blind	79	ERU	= placebo	pfr ↑ res. urine ↓	Dathe	1987	[25]
open	20	β-sitosterol	70%	pfr ↑ mv ↑ 70%	Egghart	1987	[35]
multicenter	4087	ERHU	60%	pfr ↑ res. urine ↓	Sonnenschein	1987	[72]

ERU = Extr. rad. urticae ERHU = Extr. rad. et herb. urt. mfr = mean flow rate
pfr = peak flow rate mv = micturition volume ↓ = decrease ↑ = increase

Table 3 Evaluation of phytotherapeutic drugs – controlled studies –

	agents tested	n	subj. improvement	obj. improvement	authors/ year/ref.
**	β-sitosterol vs. placebo	50 50	not recorded	better than placebo	Ebbinghaus 1977 [32]
	β-sitosterol vs. other phytopreparations	20	≈ 70%	none	Tunn 1978 [78]
*	Docosanol vs. β-sitosterol	8 8	no difference	Docosanol better than β-sitosterol clin. not relevant	Flüchter 1982 [38]
*	Docosanol vs. placebo	6 5	no difference	Docosanol better than placebo clin. not relevant	Flüchter 1982 [38]
*	Docosanol vs. ERU	15 15	not better than placebo	not significant	Schönefeld 1982 [67]
**	Docosanol vs. β-sitosterol	13 8	better than β-sitosterol	Docosanol better than placebo clin. not relevant	Walther 1982 [82]
**	ERU vs. placebo	19 22	no difference	clin. not relevant	Vontobel 1985 [80]
**	β-sitosteryl-β-D-glucoside vs. placebo	25 28	not recorded	none	Kadow 1986 [48]
	Extr. pollin. sicc. vs. β-sitosterol	19 20	better	no difference	Horvath 1986 [47]

* study performed according to FDA guidelines (1977)
** double blind study

In conclusion the use of phytotherapeutic drugs lacks scientific proof of having a causal effect on prostatic growth. There is a lot of mystics in most substances and their suggested efficacy and mode of action in BPH is poorly understood. In only a few preparations the contents are standardized. Clinical trials are controversial.

It may well be speculated whether the subjective rates of improvement might simply represent a placebo effect. Objective urodynamics according to nowadays standards have rarely been applied and in all studies even significant changes of parameters were clinically irrelevant. A real decrease in prostatic size has never been documented.

Phytotherapeutic drugs may be tried to relieve BPH-associated symptoms in stage I and II but cannot replace surgical intervention, when indicated by urodynamic criteria [37].

Organ extracts

The same critical remarks may be applied to the organ extract preparations which are suggested to increase the tone of the detrusor and improve detrusor-sphincter-dysfunction [55]. While Claridge [23] did not find a beneficial effect, others did [4, 5, 8, 24, 59]. If we look for example at the study of Albrecht [5], comparing the organ extract preparation Raveron® to sitosterol, the stated superiority of Raveron® is based on an increase of peak flow rate from 9,7 to 11,6 ml/sec after 6 months which hardly can be interpreted as a clinically relevant improvement.

The rating of residual urine in ml in this paper is inaccurate because the relation to the total voiding volume is necessary for a precise evaluation.

Problems with the evaluation of medical therapy in BPH

The analysis of a great number of controversial reports on the effect of nonhormonal treatment in BPH clearly shows the problems which are associated with a critical evaluation.

The matter is complicated by the fact that the cause of BPH is still unknown and that there is no animal model comparable to human BPH.

Several authors who have followed patients without any treatment have stressed the fluctuating character of BPH with spontaneous improvements, stable periods and deteriorations of signs and symptoms [13, 23].

Subjective symptoms can only be used as criteria when they are clearly defined and quantified by an appropriate score system, as proposed by the FDA guidelines [13].

As demonstrated in several studies a placebo effect of 40–60% has to be taken into account. It must be realized that any drug which is given to a patient with BPH, making him hope that he could possibly escape an operative intervention has an enormous placebo effect.

In order to conclude a significant subjective difference the improvement reached by a drug should at least be 75% higher than the effect reached by a placebo.

Objective parameters can only be obtained if modern urodynamic technologies and evaluations are applied. Moreover, the different urodynamic situations in patients with BPH have to be recognized. At least three different situations with regard to the detrusor function are possible: For the group of patients with obstruction and compensated detrusor function the peak flow rate (instead of mean flow rate), adjusted to the voided volume and the detrusor pressure, are necessary examinations to evaluate effects of medical therapy [29, 52, 71].

In the group of patients with residual urine, due to decompensation of the detrusor, in addition, residual urine must be calculated in relation to bladder capacity.

As patients with BPH in up to 80% show an associated detrusor hyperactivity ("instable bladder"), which in most of the patients is solely responsible for the symptoms of frequency, urgency and nocturia, detrusor reactivity has to be examined by filling cystometry. Moreover, in these patients the bladder capacity is an important parameter. It has to be taken into account that – according to Turner-Warwick [79] – the natural incidence of detrusor hyperactivity is about 25% in this age group of non obstructed men.

Changes of the detrusor reaction in correlation to flow reflect the degree of any obstruction much better than flowmetry alone. It is important that all urodynamic examinations be standardized and measured repeatedly if they should be used as objective criteria. Of course some of them are invasive and time – consuming making any clinical trial difficult for the patient and the investigator.

Even if statistical differences of objective parameters are obtained they are only of value for a patient if they are clinically relevant. Thus for example an increase of peak flow rate from 9 to 12 ml/sec may be statistically significant but is clinically of no benefit to the patient!

And finally, in the evaluation of medical therapy there is no more place for uncontrolled studies and all trials should be at least of 6 months duration to allow changes to take place.

As long as studies not satisfying these needs are still lacking and as long as trials do not prove the contrary by solid data it will be difficult to make objections to the statements of some authors like P. C. Walsh: "... in summary, there has been no controlled study of any drug that has demonstrated a meaningful improvement in patient with obstructive BPH" [81] or even to the German drug prescription report of 1987: "The numerous extracts from plants and preparations containing β-sitosterol which are offered for the treatment of incipient BPH can only be regarded as relative expensive placebos ..." [65].

References

[1] Abrams, P. H., P. J. R. Shah, R. Stone et al.: Bladder outflow obstruction treated with phenoxybenzamine. Brit. J. Urol. *54* (1982) 527–530.

[2] Abrams, P. H.: A double-blind trial of the effects of candicidin on patients with benign prostatic hypertrophy. Brit. J. Urol. *49* (1977) 67–71.

[3] Abrams, P. H., D. J. Farrar, R. T. Turner-Warwick: The results of prostatectomy: A symptomatic and urodynamic analysis of 152 patients. J. Urol. *121* (1979) 640–642.

[4] Albrecht, J.: Prostata-Adenom: Der erste Schritt ist konservativ. Ärztl Pr. *33* (1981) 2621–2622.

[5] Albrecht, J., R. Woldrich, W. J. Ziegler: Vergleichende konservative Therapie der benignen Prostatahyperplasie (BPH) mit Raveron® versus Sitosterin. Urologe (B) *24* (1984) 314–316.

[6] Andersen, J. T.: Detrusor hyperreflexia in benign infravesical obstruction. A cystometric study. J. Urol. *115* (1976) 532–534.

[7] Andersen, J. T., O. Jacobsen, J. Worm-Petersen et al.: Bladder function in healthy elderly males. Scand. J. Urol. Nephrol. *12* (1978) 123–127.

[8] Arduini, M., E. Trucchi: Doppelblindversuch über die therapeutischen Wirkungen von Raveron® beim Syndrom des Prostata-Adenoms Klin. Urol. *24* (1972) 167.

[9] Bach, D., H. Walker: How important are prostaglandins in the urology of man? Urol. Int. *37* (1982) 160–171.

[10] Böcking, A., R. Daniel: Zytologie als Verlaufskontrolle der BPH? Niere, Blase, Prostata akt. *11* (1986) 11–12.

[11] Bödeker, J., S. A. Salim, R. Nagel: Wirkungen von Nifedipin bei urologischen Patienten. DMW *101* (1976) 1866–1868.

[12] Boreham, P. F., P. Braithwaite, P. Milewski et al.: Alphaadrenergic blockers in prostatism. Br. J. Surg. *64* (1977) 756–757.

[13] Boyarsky, S., G. Jones, D. F. Paulson et al.: A new look at bladder neck obstruction by the food and drug administration regulators: Guidelines for investigators of benign prostatic hypertrophy. Transact. Am. Soc. Genit. Urin. Surg. *68* (1977) 29–32.

[14] Brandstädter, L.: Phytopharmakotherapie der benignen Prostatahyperplasie und der Prostatitis. Therapiew. *20* (1987) 1918–1923.

[15] Brooks, M. D., A. A. Sidi, Y. Hanani et al.: Ineffectiveness of phenoxybenzamine in treatment of benign prostatic hypertrophy. Urology *21* (1983) 474–478.

[16] Brühl, P.: Benigne Prostatahyperplasie (BPH). Bericht über eine Multicenterstudie zur Wirksamkeit eines β-Sitosterins. Therapiew. *35* (1985) 3629–3637.

[17] Caine, M.: The present role of alpha-adrenergic blockers in the treatment of benign prostatic hypertrophy. J. Urol. *136* (1986) 1–4.

[18] Caine, M., S. Perlberg, A. Shapiro: Phenoxybenzamine for benign prostatic obstruction. Urology *6* (1981) 542–546.

[19] Caine, M., B. Mazouz, B. M. Rossini: The effect of nicergoline on the lower urinary tract muscle. Urol. Res. *12* (1984) 287–290.

[20] Caine, M., S. Perlberg, S. Meretyk: A placebo-controlled double-blind study of the effect of phenoxybenzamine in benign prostatic obstruction. Brit. J. Urol. *50* (1978) 551–554.

[21] Caine, M., S. Raz, M. Ziegler: Adrenergic and cholinergic receptors in the human prostate, prostatic capsule and bladder neck. Brit. J. Urol. *47* (1975) 193–202.

[22] Castro, J. E.: Trial designs. Proc. roy. Soc. Med. *65* (1972) 126–127.

[23] Claridge, M.: Assessment of medical treatment: In: F. Hinmann, Jr. (ed.): Benign prostatic hypertrophy, pp. 308–312. Springer-Verlag, New York – Heidelberg 1983.

[24] Dannenberg, M., K. Weigner: Ein Therapieversuch mit Raveron® bei Männern mit Prostatahyperplasie. Urologe (B) *26* (1986) 277–279.
[25] Dathe, G., H. Schmidt: Phytotherapie der benignen Prostatahyperplasie (BPH). Urologe (B) *27* (1987) 223–226.
[26] de Klerk, D. P.: Human trials of endocrine management. In: F. Hinmann, Jr. (ed.): Benign prostatic hypertrophy, pp. 262–270. Springer-Verlag, New York–Heidelberg–Berlin 1983.
[27] Djulepa, J.: Konservative Therapie der Prostatahyperplasie bei Harnverhaltung. Med. Welt *34* (1983) 1377–1379.
[28] Djulepa, J.: Zweijährige Erfahrung in der Therapie des Prostata-Syndroms. Ärztl. Praxis *63* (1982) 2199.
[29] Drach, G. W., W. Binard: Disposable peak urinary flowmeter estimates lower urinary tract obstruction. J. Urol. *115* (1976) 175–179.
[30] Dreßler, H.: Therapeutische Erfahrungen mit β-Sitosterin (Prostasal®) zur konservativen Behandlung des Prostata-Adenoms. Extr. Urol. *6* (1983) 364–372.
[31] Ebbinghaus, K. D.: Die konservative Therapie des Prostata-Adenoms. MMW *50* (1974) 2209–2212.
[32] Ebbinghaus, K. D., M. P. Baur: Ergebnisse einer Doppelblindstudie über die Wirksamkeit eines Medikamentes zur konservativen Behandlung des Prostata-Adenoms. Z. Allg. Med. *53* (1977) 1054–1058.
[33] Ebers: Papyrus discovered at Luxor Cited by Edwards, L. 1872.
[34] Edwards, L.: History of nonsurgical treatment. In: F. Hinman, Jr. (ed.): Benign prostatic hypertrophy, pp. 30–34. Springer-Verlag, New York–Heidelberg–Berlin 1983.
[35] Egghart, G., F. Gallyas: Klinische Erfahrungen mit Harzol®-Kapseln in der Behandlung des Prostata-Adenoms. Urologe (B) *27* (1987) 227–231.
[36] Ferrie, B. G., P. J. Paterson: Phenoxybenzamine in prostatic hypertrophy, a doubleblind study. Brit. J. Urol. *59* (1987) 63–65.
[37] Flamm, J., H. Kiesswetter, M.: Urodynamische Verlaufskontrolle bei konservativer Behandlung des Prostata-Adenoms mit Phytopräparat und Testosteron. Wien. Klin. Wschr. *91* (1979) 622–627.
[38] Flüchter, St. H., K.-H. Bichler, R. Harzmann et al.: Konservative Therapie des Prostataadenoms mit Docosanol. Ergebnisse zweier Doppelblindprüfungen. Klin. Exp. Urol. *4* (1982) 165–172.
[39] Forman, A., K.-E. Andersson, L. Henriksson et al.: Effects of nifedipine on the smooth muscle of the human urinary tract in vitro and in vivo. Acta pharmcol. et toxicol. *43* (1978) 111–118.
[40] Furuya, S., Y. Kumamoto, E. Yokoyama et al.: Alpha-adrenergic activity and urethral pressure in prostatic zone in benign prostatic hypertrophy. J. Urol. *128* (1982) 836–839.
[41] Gerstenberg, T., J. Blaabbjerg, M. Lykkegaard et al.: Phenoxybenzamine reduces bladder outlet obstruction in benign prostatic hyperplasia. Invest. Urol. *18* (1980) 29–31.
[42] Goldstein, N. I.: Cholesterol synthesis in the prostate gland and its relationship to benign prostatic hyperplasia. In: PhD dissertation, Rutgers University, New Brunswick, New York 1975.
[43] Gordon, H. W., C. P. Schaffner: The effect of polyene macrolides on the prostate gland and canine prostatic hyperplasia. Proc. Natl. Acad. Sci. USA *60* (1968) 1201–1208.
[44] Gupta, M. B., R. Nath, N. Srivastava et al.: Anti-inflammatory and antipyretic activities of β-sitosterol. Planta med. *39* (1980) 157–163.
[45] Hedlund, H., K. E. Andersson, A. Ek: Effects of prazosin in patients with benign prostatic obstruction. J. Urol. *130* (1983) 275–278.

[46] Henneking, K., H. Heckers: Prostataadenom. Indikation zur Therapie mit sitosterinhaltigen Phytopharmaka. Med. Welt *34* (1983) 625–632.

[47] Horvath, L., H. Bräuer, K. Scheffer et al.: Phytopharmaka-Therapie der benignen Prostatahyperplasie. Therapiew. *36* (1986) 1686–1696.

[48] Kadow, C., P. H. Abrams: A double-blind trial of the effect of beta-sitosteryl glucoside (WA 184) in the treatment of benign prostatic hyperplasia. Eur. Urol. *12* (1986) 187–189.

[49] Keshin, J. G.: Effect of candicidin on the human benign hypertrophied prostate gland. Int. Surg. *58* (1973) 116–122.

[50] Klingeberg, J.: Harnflußmessung in der Praxis. Zeitschr. Allg. Med. *57* (1981) 1934–1937.

[51] Kündig, H.: Zur Toxikologie und Pharmakologie der Sitosterin-Fraktion aus Hypoxis rooperi. Notab. Med. *9* (1981) 358–363.

[52] Layton, T. N., G. W. Drach: Selectivity of peak versus average male urinary flow rates. J. Urol. *125* (1981) 839–841.

[53] Lukkarinen, D.: Total and SHBG-bound testosterone and 5a-Dihydrostestosterone serum concentrations in normal elderly men and patients with benign prostatic hypertrophy before and after removal of the adenoma. Brit. J. Urol. *52* (1980) 377–380.

[54] Orkin, L. A.: Efficacy of candicidin in benign prostatic hypertrophy. Urology *4* (1974) 80–84.

[55] Pegel, K. H.: β-sitosterin-β-d-glucosid (Sitosterolin). Eine aktive Wirksubstanz in Harzol. Extr. Urol. *7* (1984) 105–111.

[56] Pegel, K. H., H. Walker: Neue Aspekte zur benignen Prostata-Hyperplasie (BPH). Die Rolle der Leukotriene und Prostaglandine bei der Entstehung sowie bei der konservativen Therapie, der durch sie verursachten Symptome. Extr. Urol. *7* (1984) 91–96.

[57] Pegel, K. H., H. Walker: Phytosterol senkt mutagenes Epoxyd. Therapiew. *36* (1986) 1845–1848.

[58] Ronchi, F., A. Margonato, A. Ceccardi et al.: Symptomatic treatment of benign prostatic obstruction with nicergoline: A placebo controlled clinical study and urodynamic evaluation. Urol. Res. *10* (1982) 131–134.

[59] Rummani, F.: Zur Therapie des Prostata-Adenoms und der Prostatitis mit Harzol – statistische Auswertung einer retrospektiven Studie. Extr. Med. Pract. *2* (1981) 393–398.

[60] Rugendorff, E. W.: Therapieerfahrungen mit Raveron® bei der Behandlung der benignen Prostatahyperplasie – eine Erhebung aus 10 Arztpraxen. Ärztl. Prax. *39* (1987) 2446–2448.

[61] Schaffner, C. P.: Effect of cholesterol-lowering agents. In: F. Hinman, Jr. (ed.): Benign prostatic hypertrophy, pp. 280–312. Springer-Verlag, New York – Heidelberg – Berlin 1983.

[62] Schilcher, H., M. Sauter, H. Janssen: Zum Wirksamkeitsnachweis von Phytopharmaka am Beispiel von Prosta-Fink. Ärzteztschr. Naturheilv. *26* (1985) 175–185.

[63] Schindler, E.: Die Frühoperation des Prostataadenoms muß nicht sein. Ärztl. Prax. *35* (1983) 1717–1718.

[64] Schmidt, K.: Die Wirkung eines Radix-Urticae-Extrakts und einzelner Nebenextrakte auf das SHBG des Blutplasmas bei der benignen Prostatahyperplasie. Fortschr. Med. *101* (1983) 713–716.

[65] Schmitz, W. Urologika. In: U. Schwabe, D. Paffrath (eds): Arzneimittelverordnungs-Report 87, pp. 365–373. G. Fischer, Stuttgart – New York 1987.

[66] Schneider, H. J.: Konservative Behandlung der benignen Prostatahyperplasie (BPH). Ztschr. Allg. Med. *30* (1986) 1069–1072.

[67] Schönefeld, G., R. Tauber, U. Rattenhuber et al.: Die Bedeutung von Docosanol und Extractum Radicis Urticae zur konservativen Therapie der Prostatahyperplasie. Klin. Exp. Urol. *4* (1982) 179–182.

[68] Scott, W. W., D. S. Coffey: Nonsurgical treatment of human benign prostatic hyperplasia. Vitam. Horm. *33* (1975) 439–465.

[69] Shapiro, A., B. Mazouz, M. Caine: The alpha-adrenergic blocking effect of prazosin on the human prostate. Urol. Res. *9* (1987) 17–20.

[70] Singhard, A. K., D. P. Bonner, C. P. Schaffner: Kinetics of testosterone induced – cholesterol synthesis in rat ventral prostate. Proc. Soc. Exp. Biol. Med. *159* (1975) 1–5.

[71] Siroky, M. B., C. A. Olson, R. J. Krane: The flow rate nomogramm: I. development. J. Urol. *122* (1979) 665–668.

[72] Sonnenschein, R.: Untersuchung der Wirksamkeit eines prostatotrophen Phytotherapeutikums (Urtica plus) bei benigner Prostatahyperplasie und Prostatitis – eine prospektive multizentrische Studie. Urologe (B) 27 (1987) 231–237.

[73] Sporer, A., S. Cohen, M. H. Kamat: Candicidin: Physiologic effect on prostate. Urology 6 (1975) 298–304.

[74] Stahl, H.-P.: Die Therapie prostatischer Nykturie. Ztschr. Allg. Med. *60* (1984) 128–132.

[75] Streber, A. S.: Künftig mit Pseudo-Testosteron gegen Prostata-Adenom? Ärztl. Prax. *28* (1981) 1045–1047.

[76] Swyer, G. I. M.: The cholesterol content of normal and enlarged prostates. Cancer Res. (1942) 372–375.

[77] Tosch, U., H. Müssiggang: Medikamentöse Behandlung der benignen Prostatahyperplasie. Euromed 6 (1983).

[78] Tunn, U., Th. Senge: Untersuchungen zum Wirkungserfolg der konservativen Behandlung bei benigner Prostatahyperplasie durch Uroflowmetrie. Z. Urol. u. Nephrol. *71* (1978) 521–528.

[79] Turner-Warwick, R.: Bladder outflow obstruction in the male. In: A. R. Munday, T. P. Stephenson, A. J. Wein (eds): Urodynamics, pp. 183–204. Churchill Livingsstone, Edinbourgh – London 1984.

[80] Vontobel, H. P., R. Herzog, G. Rutishauser et al.: Ergebnisse einer Doppelblindstudie über die Wirksamkeit von ERU-Kapseln in der konservativen Behandlung der benignen Prostatahyperplasie. Urologe (A) *24* (1985) 49–51.

[81] Walsh, P. C.: Benign prostatic hyperplasia. In: P. C. Walsh, R. F. Gittes, A. D. Perlmutter (eds): Campbell's Urology, pp. 1247–1265. W. B. Saunders, Philadelphia, 1986.

[82] Walther, V., G. Stachler, J. Schüller et al.: Ergebnisse einer Doppelblindstudie über die Wirksamkeit von Docosanol und β-Sitosterin zur konservativen Behandlung des Prostataadenoms. Klin. Exp. Urol. *4* (1982) 173–178.

[83] Zahradnik, H. P., R. Schillfahrt, R. Schoening et al.: Prostaglandin-Gehalt in Prostata-Adenomen nach Behandlung mit einem Sterol. Fortschr. Med. *98* (1980) 69–72.

[84] Ziegler, H.: Zytomorphologische Untersuchungen der benignen Prostatahyperplasie unter Behandlung mit Extract. Radicis Urticae (ERU). Fortschr. Med. *39* (1982) 1832–1834.

Management of benign prostatic hyperplasia with antiandrogens and antiestrogens – clinical results (Review)

R. Tenaglia, F. Di Silverio

Introduction

In 1896, Cabot suggested the first use of hormonal therapy with castration [2]. Since then, there have been several attempts at hormonal therapy of BPH. In recent times the remarkable improvement achieved by research has allowed the establishment of a rational basis for a "casual" treatment.

Age related alterations of the hormonal balance, morphogenesis of BPH, and interaction between stroma and prostatic epithelium related to the mechanism of endocrine regulations have been documented.

In 1979, supported by the information gathered from several authors and particularly from experimentation on animal models, we started to treat patients afflicted with noncomplicated BPH with the antiandrogen cyproterone acetate (CA) and with the antiestrogen tamoxifen (TAM).

Here we shall present the rationale that has directed us towards this hormonal therapy as well as the experience we acquired with this concept.

Materials and methods

Since 1979, over 500 patients have been treated with CA in combination with TAM. The findings presented in this article refer to a randomized trial started in 1983. The study was done on a group of 256 patients with the aim of comparing therapy effects of gestonorone caproate (GC), of CA and of CA plus TAM [4]. Prerequisites for the patients were: noncomplicated BPH, no hepatic or renal insufficiencies and no previous treatment.

Number and mean age of patients as well as length of treatment are shown on table 1.

New Developments in Biosciences 5

Table 1 Data on 3 study groups

Treatment			
	GC (200 mg/week)	CA (50 mg/day)	CA* + TAM** (50* + 20** mg/day)
Patients (n)	90	83	83
Mean age (years)	68.1	66.9	68.2

Treatment period = 2 months
GC = 200 mg/week
CA = 50 mg/day
CA* + TAM** = 50* + 20** mg/day

Table 2 Clinical parameters

A. Subjective
- nycturia, daytime frequency, urgency, incontinence, end of dripping, free interval time, waiting time, bladder emptying, continuous flow, potency.

B. Objective
- prostatic diameters (with transrectal ultrasounds): longitudinal (LD), transversal (TD), anteroposterior (APD).
- prostatic volume (cmc) $= 4/3\,\pi \frac{LD \cdot TD \cdot APD}{2}$
- postmictional residue (with suprapubic U.S.)
- uroflow

The assessed clinical parameters are shown in table 2. The clinical findings have been classified within three categories of responses: improvement (I), worsening (W), no change (NC). In addition, serum concentrations for testosterone, FSH, LH and prolactin (PRL) were determined for the group treated with CA plus TAM both before and after treatment.

Results

Significant differences were not noticed among the three groups with regard to the following subjective parameter: incontinence, terminal dripping, potency, urgency, waiting time. The highest improvement in nycturia (table 3), voiding frequency (table 4) and incomplete bladder emptying (table 5) was observed in the group of patients treated with CA plus TAM as compared to those treated with GC and CA alone. With regard to the objective parameters, the most notable variations were observed between the group treated with CA plus TAM and the two other groups in regard to the prostate volume (table 6), the post-mictional residual urine (table 7) and the urinary flow (table 8). The mean values of testosterone, FSH, LH and PRL noted before and after treatment with CA plus TAM are shown on table 9. PRL increased slightly.

Table 3 Nycturia

Response	GC		CA		CA + TAM	
	n	%	n	%	n	%
I	39	47	28	35.5	48	60
NC	42	50.6	48	60.7	31	38.7
W	2	2.4	3	3.8	1	1.3

Table 4 Daytime frequency

Response	GC		CA		CA + TAM	
	n	%	n	%	n	%
I	34	40.5	38	47.5	52	65
NC	44	52.4	37	46.3	25	31.3
W	6	7.1	5	6.2	3	3.7

Table 5 Bladder never empty

Response	GC		CA		CA + TAM	
	n	%	n	%	n	%
I	21	43.7	25	58	32	64
NC	25	52.1	20	40	17	34
W	2	4.2	1	2	1	2

Table 6 Prostate volume

Response	GC		CA		CA + TAM	
	n	%	n	%	n	%
I	23	28.7	23	29.8	44	55
NC	57	71.3	54	70.2	36	45
W	0	0	0	0	0	0

Table 7 Post-mictional residue

Response	GC		CA		CA + TAM	
	n	%	n	%	n	%
I	36	45	32	40	56	70
NC	40	50	42	52.5	24	30
W	4	5	6	7.5	0	0

Table 8 Urinary flow

Response	GC		CA		CA + TAM	
	n	%	n	%	n	%
I	22	28.6	27	36	36	46.2
NC	55	71.4	48	64	42	53.8
W	0	0	0	0	0	0

Table 9 Testosterone, LH, FSH and PRL-plasma value before and after treatment with CA + TAM

Hormone		Basal	After treatment
Testosterone	(ng/ml)	3.22	3.25
LS	(mlU/ml)	10.32	12.15
FSH	(mlU/ml)	9.58	8.57
PRL	(mg/ml)	8.28	11.05

Discussion

The principal considerations for a treatment of BPH with antiandrogens plus antiestrogens are listed in table 10. Morphological alterations are seen in 8% of 30–40 years old men and are found in 60–70% of those of 70 years of age [13].

Table 10 Rationale for treatment of BPH with antiandrogens plus antiestrogens

1. Age-related alterations of blood hormonal values
2. Origin and evolution of BPH
3. Hormonal regulation of stroma and epithelium and their interactions-stereology
4. Experimentally induced BPH and its inhibition

Several endocrine alterations which reduce the relationship between free testosterone and free estrogens have been documented in patients of about 60 years of age [15]. These variations may stimulate proliferation capacities of the embryonal type in some prostatic areas. As documented by McNeal [10] and Pradhan [13], the transition area and the periurethral stroma are the privileged sites where starting stromal nodules appear. Their histological appearance clearly resembles the embryonal mesenchyme. It can be demonstrated on serial sections of the prostate taken from subjects of various ages that such nodules appear spontaneously in a focal manner in patients under the age of forty [10] and increase in volume due to a hormonal imbalance which appears around the age of sixty. This corresponds to a rapid hypertrophy of both stromal and particularly of epithelial elements. Numerous authors [8, 12, 14] have verified the preferential binding of the estrogens in the stroma of the BPH because of the presence of specific receptors, and their activity on the formation of hyperplasia. The stroma itself exerts on the epithelium not only a function of support, but also of induction and modulation of growth [3, 11]. This is due to the presence of the 5-α-reductase which catalizes the transformation of testosterone into dihydrotestosterone (DHT), the biologically active androgen [9]. Moreover, it has shown that in the stromal part of the prostate (guinea pig), the endogenous concentration of estrogens exceeds that of the plasma. These findings support the theory that endogenous estrogens may be of importance in the regulation of stromal function [1]. The role of DHT in BPH has been extensively discussed: in fact some authors seemed to have found higher concentrations in BPH than in normal prostatic tissue [6]. This finding has been refused by Walsh [16]. Current research seems to direct its attention to estrogenic stimulation of the prostatic stroma [3]. Bruchovsky [9] has noted the maximum activity level of 5-α-reductase within the stromal compartment, a phenomenon even more evident in BPH.

Neumann [5] has proved on dogs that androgens stimulate mainly the epithelium, while estrogens induce in particular the stimulation of the stroma. In addition, such effects are antagonized by the contemporary administration of antiandrogens (CA) and antiestrogens (TAM). Since the TAM is not a pure antiestrogen, Habenicht et al. [7] have achieved much more specific antiestrogenic effects utilizing an aromatase inhibitor. Findings described by Neumann made up the basis of our clinical experience.

Hormonal therapy may possibly be the only means of “casual” treatment of BPH. Hormonal therapy has its place in cases of patients having low-middle grade symptoms or patients who refuse, wish to postpone or cannot face surgery because of general contraindications.

Still much has to be done to improve the results and to reduce side effects (78% of our patients showed libido decrease). Making antiestrogenic effects more selective is also important.

The TAM has not been used separately in this trial because of the well-known stimulation effects of gonadotropins and subsequent testosterone increase. In fact, after stimulation of the hypothalamic-pituitary-gonadal axis by administration of TAM, the fine structure of the ventral prostatic gland of the rat is morphologically similar to that of adult male rats after treatment with high dosage of testosterone. The stereological data suggests a proliferation of glandular epithelium [1]. In conclusion, more knowledge is required of estrogenic as well as antiestrogenic effects of TAM. In the meantime drugs with true antiestrogenic effects should be tested for their therapeutic value in this disease.

References

[1] Bartsch, G., H. Rohr: Stereology – A new method to assess normal and pathological growth of the prostate. In: G. H. Jacobi, R. Hohenfellner (eds): Prostate Cancer, p. 433. Williams & Wilkins, Baltimore 1982.

[2] Cabot, W.: The question of castration for enlarged prostate. Ann. Surg. Phila *165* (1896).

[3] Cunha, G. R., B. Lung: The importance of stroma in morphogenesis and functional activity of urogenital epithelium. In Vitro *15* (1979) 50.

[4] Di Silverio, F., R. Tenaglia: Antiestrogens and antiandrogens in human benign prostatic hyperplasia. In: F. Di Silverio, F. Neumann, M. Tannenbaum (eds): Ipertrofia prostatica benigna – Atti del Simposio Internazionale. Taormina, Ottobre 1985. Excerpta Medica, Amsterdam 1986.

[5] Funke, P. J., U. W. Tunn, T. Sence et al.: Histological and histochemical findings in prostates of castrated dogs after treatment with estradiol, tamoxifen, androstanediol and cyproterone acetate. In: J. E. Altwein, G. Bartsch, G. H. Jacobi (eds): Antihormone – Bedeutung in der Urologie, p. 51. W. Zuckerschwerdt Verlag, Munich 1981.

[6] Geller, J., J. Albert, D. Lopez et al.: Comparison of androgen metabolites in benign prostatic hypertrophy (BPH) and normal prostate. J. Clin. Endocrinol. Metab. *43* (1976) 686.

[7] Habenicht, U. F., K. Schwarz, H. U. Schweikert et al.: Development of a model for the introduction of estrogen – related prostatic hyperplasia in the dog and its response to the aromatase inhibitor 4-hydroxy-4-androstene-3,17-dione. Prostate *8* (1985) 181.

[8] Krieg, M., G. Klötzl, J. Kaufmann et al.: Stroma of human benign prostatic hyperplasia: prefential tissue for androgen metabolism and estrogen binding. Acta Endocrinol. *96* (1981) 422.

[9] McLoughlin, M. G., N. Bruchovsky: Stromal-Epithelial interaction. In: F. Hinman, Jr. (ed.): Benign Prostatic Hypertrophy, p. 130. Springer-Verlag, New York 1983.

[10] McNeal, J. E.: Relationship of the origin of benign prostatic hypertrophy to prostatic structure of man and other mammals. In: F. Hinman, Jr. (ed.): Benign Prostatic hypertrophy, p. 152. Springer-Verlag, New York 1983.

[11] Muntzing, J., J. Liljekist, G. P. Murphy: Chalones and stroma as possible growth-limiting factors in the rat ventral prostate. Invest. Urol. *16* (1979) 399.

[12] Murphy, J. B., R. C. Emmott, L. L. Hicks et al.: Estrogen receptors in the human prostate, seminal vesicles epididymis, testis, and genital skin: a marker for estrogen-responsive tissue? J. Clin. Endocrinal. Metab. *50* (1980) 838.

[13] Pradham, B. K., K. Chandra: Morphogenesis of nodular hyperplasia-prostate. J. Urol. *113* (1975) 210.
[14] Thompson, S. A., D. R. Rowley, P. M. Heidger, Jr.: Effects of estrogen upon the fine structures epithelium and stroma in the rat ventral prostate gland. Invest. Urol *17* (1979) 83.
[15] Vermeulen, A.: Testicular hormonal secretion and aging in mammals. In: J. T. Grayack, J. D. Wilson, M. J. Scherbenske (eds): Benign prostatic hyperplasia, p. 177. DHEW Publication (NIH), Washington 1975.
[16] Walsh, P. C., G. M. Hutchins, L. L. Ewing: Tissue content of dihydrotestosterone in human prostatic hyperplasia is not supranormal. J. Clin. Invest. 72 (1983) 1772.

Androgen ablation in the treatment of stage II benign prostatic hyperplasia

F. H. Schröder, R. J. L. H. Bosch, J. H. M. Blom

Androgen dependence of BPH

The morphogenesis of the normal prostate during embryonal and puberal life is governed by androgens. In the absence of androgens or in the absence of mechanisms that allow circulating androgens to act at the target cell like in the syndrom of testicular feminization together with other secondary male characteristic the prostate does not develop.

The question whether the pathogenesis of human prostatic tumors, namely prostatic cancer and benign prostatic hyperplasia (BPH) is regulated by androgens has been under discussion for almost 100 years and is still not resolved. The British surgeon White reported in 1895 [10] rapid atrophy of the prostate with improvement of micturition in 87.2% of 111 cases treated by castration. Cabot, in 1896 [2] stated about 79 cases who survived bilateral castration that chronic retention, which was present in 27 of these patients, subsided after castration. He felt that substantial improvement was seen in 83.6% of his patient population. Both authors did not differentiate between enlargement of the prostate due to carcinoma and BPH.

The fact that androgen receptors are present in epithelium and stroma of BPH and that androgen metabolism takes place in the same tissue compartments, strongly suggests that androgens play a role in the growth and maintenance of this tumor. Huggins and Stevens [4] showed as early as 1940 in 3 patients with BPH, who underwent prostatectomy after castration, that atrophy mainly of the epithelial part results from androgen ablation. This was confirmed by Wendel et al. in 1972 [9].

Besides androgen ablation other modalities of treatment like the combination of androgen ablation with an anti-estrogen [3] and the application of an aromatase inhibitor was studied in BPH patients. These studies, also of importance in the whole context of the issue of conservative management of BPH, will not be considered in this chapter dealing only with androgen ablation.

At the Department of Urology, Erasmus University Rotterdam, The Netherlands, two studies have been carried out in recent years in which androgen ablation is

New Developments in Biosciences 5

applied to patients suffering from BPH. In study I patients suffering from stage III BPH disease (chronic urinary retention with indwelling catheters) who were in too poor a general condition for undergoing surgery were selected. In study II patients suffering from stage II symptomatic BPH were included. Both studies have been previously published [1, 6] but will be summarized and discussed in this chapter.

A study of androgen ablation in 6 patients with BPH stage III

In this first study, which was carried out during the years from 1977 through 1985, 6 patients were selected for androgen ablation treatment. All patients suffered from stage III BPH with chronic urinary retention necessitating indwelling catheter treatment. Because of poor general condition usually due to cardiac failure and cardiac ischemia, surgery by means of transurethral or open prostatectomy was impossible. Prostatic volumes measured by transrectal ultrasound prior to treatment averaged 76.4 cm^3 with a range of 38 – 96 cm^3. Five patients were treated by means of castration under local anesthesia, one patient, who went into chronic urinary retention just after a myocardial infarction with development of a left ventricular aneurysm was treated by means of the LHRH analogue Busereline, 0.4 mg intranassaly t.i.d. All patients except one who refused were followed by regular 1 – 2 monthly measurements of their prostatic volume by means of transrectal ultrasonography.

Results

Results are summarized in table 1. All patients showed a dramatic decrease of prostatic volume after 2 – 3 months. The volume reduction averaged 31.4% with a range of 19 – 55%. All patients were able to void after 2 – 5 months and continued to do so for an average of 11.2 months of follow-up. In the patient who was treated by means of the LHRH analogue prostatic volume increased

Table 1 Study I – results of androgen ablation in 6 patients with stage III BPH [6]

- All patients showed a prostatic volume decrease after 2 – 3 months
- The volume reduction averaged 31.4% (19 – 55%)
- All patients were able to void after 2 – 5 months and continued to do so for an average of 11.2 months of follow-up
- After discontinuation of LHRH BPH recurred

after the discontinuation of treatment. All previous symptoms including chronic urinary retention recurred. Residual urine disappeared completely in 5 of the 6 patients. One patient kept on retaining some urine but was able to urinate freely and did not require a catheter anymore.

The loss of potency associated with castration or LHRH management was not studied in this particular series of patients because it was of no concern from the beginning on.

Androgen withdrawal in 12 patients with BPH stage II

Into this second study 12 patients with obstructive symptoms and an enlarged benign prostate were included. Prior to entry patients were extensively informed about the studies included in this protocol, especially about the transrectal ultrasonography and repeated urodynamic evaluation. Only patients who were willing to sign an informed consent after this conversation were included. In addition to clinical signs and symptoms there also had to be urodynamic evidence of obstruction mainly by means of evaluation of a pressure flow plot. It was interesting to see that of 18 patients who were considered to have obstructive BPH on clinical grounds only 12 qualified by means of their urodynamic studies. All patients had residual urine above 50 cm^3, average prostatic volume prior to entry was found to be 41 ml with a range of 15 – 83 ml.

Treatment

Patients were randomly assigned to 12 weeks of treatment with Cyproterone acetate or to LHRH (Busereline) application. The Busereline group had to be pretreated and patients were entered into the trial at the moment that their plasma testosterone had reached castration level. This point in time was considered week 0. Pretreatment periods ranged between 2 and 4 weeks. Cyproterone acetate (CPA) 100 mg was given orally b.i.d. Busereline was applied intranasally in a dosage of 0.4 mg t.i.d. Treatment was discontinued at 12 weeks, the trial period lasted 24 weeks.

Methods

Besides the regular routine clinical examinations the patients were requested to fill in micturition diary cards to record the daily and nightly frequency of urination. Prostatic volume was measured by means of transrectal ultrasonography at time 0 and then in 2–4-weekly intervals. Video urodynamic studies were carried out at time 0, 6, 12 and 24 weeks. The urodynamic studies included the determination of the maximal flow rate, the peak detrusor pressure, the maximum detrusor contraction strength and other parameters. Statistical examination was carried out by variance analysis, Wilcoxon's matched pair signed ranks test and Spearmans rank correlation coefficient. The treatment and evaluation scheme is depicted in table 2.

Table 2 Study II – treatment scheme [1]

Week	Treatment	Studies
2 to 3	start LHRH	pre-study evaluation
0	start CPA	–
6	continue	U.S. + urodyn.
12	stop	U.S. + urodyn.
24	none	U.S. + urodyn.

Off-study patients

Of 18 patients with clinical signs and symptoms of BPH only 12 qualified for the study on the basis of the urodynamic parameters for obstruction used. In the Busereline group one patient did not reach castration levels of plasma testosterone, 2 patients discontinued treatment. In the CPA group one patient suffered a CVA after 9 weeks, another patient continued treatment beyond 12 weeks.

Results, study II

Prostatic volumes decreased significantly after 6 weeks as compared to prostatic volume at entry into the study. The further decrease between 6 and 12 weeks was not significant. The volume increase found after discontinuation of treatment at week 24 was significant as compared to the volumes found at week 12. These data are summarized in table 3.

The frequency of urination was significantly improved during daytime at week 12. No night time improvement was seen. After 24 weeks the improvement seen at week 12 had for some part disappeared. In absolute numbers the difference observed in daytime voiding frequency amounts to a decrease of 8.3 to 7.0 times at 12 weeks. Obviously, in spite of statistical significance very little clinical significance can be attributed to this finding. The data are summarized in table 4.

Table 3 Study II – prostatic volumes n = 12 [1]

Week	Nr. pts.	Volume (%)
0	12	100
6	11*	76.5
12	10*	70.8
24	7**	97.0

Prostatic volumes week 0: $\bar{x}$ = 41 ml (15 – 83 ml)
* $p < 0.005$ (compared to week 0)
** $p < 0.01$ (compared to week 12)

Table 4 Study II – frequency of urination [1]

Week	N	Day ($\bar{x}$)	Night ($\bar{x}$)
0	8	8.3	1.9
6	8	8.1	2.2
12	8	7.0*	1.9
24	7	7.4	1.7

* $p < 0.025$ compared to week 0

Table 5 Study I – urodynamic findings [1]

- Detrusor pressure at peak flow, effective urethral caliber (FGU), urethral resistance (URA), prostatic plateau length – not significant
- Maximum flow rate: week 0 – 9.6 ml/sec
  week 12 – 10.6 ml/sec, $p < 0.025$
- Residual urine: week 0 – 50.9 ml
  week 12 – 34.9 ml, $p < 0.05$
- Detrusor contraction strength (W max): week 6 – 9.7 uW/mm^2
  week 12 – 10.6 uW/mm^2, $p < 0.025$

The urodynamic findings also produced some statistically significant results of questionable clinical importance. The data are summarized in table 5.

There was an improvement of the maximal flow rate from 9.6 ml/sec at week 0 to 10.6 ml/sec at week 12. This was significant with a p value < 0.025. The residual urine decreased from week 2 – 12 from an average of 50.9 to 34.9 ml. This was different at a p value < 0.05. Detrusor contraction strength (Wmax) also improved significantly between week 6 and 12 without amounting to clinical relevance. There was an impression, that the urodynamic improvements did not parallel the volume changes of the prostate but were delayed. The possibility that with continuation of treatment beyond the period of 3 months further improvement could have been obtained cannot be excluded.

Side effects

Hot flushes and impotence were the major side effects occurring in both arms of the study. Two of six CPA patients and all Busereline patients suffered of hot flushes. In the CPA group one cerebrovascular accident occurred after 9 weeks. The question whether this is attributable to the CPA treatment cannot be resolved. Seven of the twelve patients claimed at entry to be potent and sexually active. All except one CPA patient became impotent during the study and in all except one LHRH patients potency reoccurred after varying periods of time after discontinuation of treatment. The one patient who still remains sexually inactive after LHRH treatment underwent a TUR prostate in the meantime and is expected to become potent after complete recovery.

Conclusions and discussion

By means of androgen withdrawal a significant reduction of prostatic volume in BPH patients can be achieved within 6 weeks. The average of 36% volume decrease seems to be independent of the original volume and was remarkably similar in another study of BPH patients treated with the LHRH analogue Nafarelin by Peters et al. [5]. These authors have also confirmed by biopsy and morphometry that the volume reduction is mainly due to a decrease of the epithelial fraction of the BPH specimens. Prostatic volume reduction reverses after discontinuation of treatment, the increase of prostatic volume is associated with a return of the original symptoms especially in the group of patients who were suffering from chronic urinary retention (stage III BPH).

In 6 patients suffering from chronic urinary retention due to BPH a dramatic clinical improvement occurred. In all patients the prostatic volume reduction was paralleled by the return of the ability to urinate and the possibility to discontinue longstanding indwelling catheter treatment.

In the clinically symptomatic patients who all showed a clear cut indication for transurethral resection in study II the prostatic volume reduction was not associated with a dramatic clinical improvement. The numerically significant improvements of the rate of micturition, maximal urinary flow rate and some other urodynamic parameters, is clinically not very meaningful.

Impotence and hot flushes were side effects in many patients of study II. These side effects are not acceptable in a situation were transurethral resection or open prostatectomy will remain the first treatment option. However, if new principles of treatment such as aromatase inhibition and 5-alpha-reductase inhibition could produce prostatic volume reduction and at the same time maintenance of potency, the principle of intraprostatic counteraction of steroidal growth stimuli could result in conservative management of BPH.

References

[1] Bosch, J. L. H., D. J. Griffiths, J. H. M. Blom et al.: Treatment of benign prostatic hyperplasia by androgen deprivation: effects on prostate size and urodynamic parameters. J. Urol. *141* (1989) 68 – 72.

[2] Cabot, A. T.: The question of castration for enlarged prostate. Ann. Surg. *24* (1896) 265 – 309.

[3] Di Silverio, F., R. Tenaglia: Anti-estrogens and anti-androgens in human benign prostatic hyperplasia. In: F. Di Silverio, F. Neumann, M. Tannenbaum (eds): Ipertrofia prostatica benigna, pp. 117 – 125. Excerpta Medica, Amsterdam – Sydney – Tokyo 1986.

[4] Huggins, C., R. Stevens: The effect of castration on benign hypertrophy of the prostate in man. J. Urol. *43* (1940) 705 – 714.

[5] Peters, C. A., P. C. Walsh: The effect of nafarelin acetate, a luiteinizing-hormone-releasing hormone agonist on benign prostatic hyperplasia. New Engl. J. Med. *317* (1987) 599 – 604.

[6] Schröder, F. H., M. Westerhof, R. J. L. H. Bosch et al.: Benign prostatic hyperplasia treated by castration or the LHRH analogue Busereline: a report on 6 cases. Eur. Urol. *12* (1986) 318 – 321.

[7] Scott, W. W.: What makes the prostate grow? J. Urol. *70* (1953) 477 – 488.

[8] Tunn, U. W., P. Kaivers, H. U. Schweikert: Conservative treatment of human prostatic hyperplasia. In: N. Bruchorsky, A. Chapdelaine, F. Neumann (eds): Regulation of androgen action. R. Brückner, Berlin 1985.

[9] Wendel, E. F., G. E. Brannen, P. B. Putong et al.: The effect of orchiectomy and estrogens on benign prostatic hyperplasia. J. Urol. *198* (1972) 116 – 119.

[10] White, J. W.: The results of double castration in hypertrophy of the prostate. Ann. Surg. *22* (1895) 1 – 80.

Aromatase inhibitors in the management of benign prostatic hyperplasia

U. W. Tunn, H. U. Schweikert

Introduction

Prostatic disease has been haunting the male members of mankind for a long time. The attempt of aiding micturition by some kind of medication can be traced back to the 15th century b.C. An Egyptian papyros gives this prescription to relieve micturition problems: one part of junifer bark, cypress bark, and beer, the whole to be crushed, cooked and strained before drinking it over a period of four days.

The treatment of choice for voiding problems caused by benign prostatic hyperplasia (BPH) is surgical. We do not have any established pharmacological therapy. Aromatase inhibitors present a new therapeutic concept in BPH [7, 12]. In this paper our group reports the first results of aromatase inhibitors in experimental and clinical practice.

Our knowledge of etiology of BPH as well as present and future concepts of conservative therapy are discussed exhaustingly in other chapters of this book. In summary, onset and maintenance of BPH must be regarded as an endocrinopathy. Androgens and estrogens seem to have a pacemaker function [3, 13].

In summary, active steroids will be created and bind themselves to androgen and estrogen receptors with varying affinity and will trigger protein synthesis and cell replication in stroma and epithelium.

Estrogens and BPH

Many facts point to estrogens playing an important role in the pathogenesis of BPH. In this context the proven estrogen accumulation in human BPH tissue shall be underlined. According to Kozak et al. the estrone (E_1) and estradiol (E_2) content in BPH is significantly higher than in plasma with an E_2/E_1 ratio of 2.5 [4]. Estrogens were found almost exclusively in stromal nuclei and not in epithelium [5]. Stroma seems to have a key function in BPH pathogenesis.

New Developments in Biosciences 5

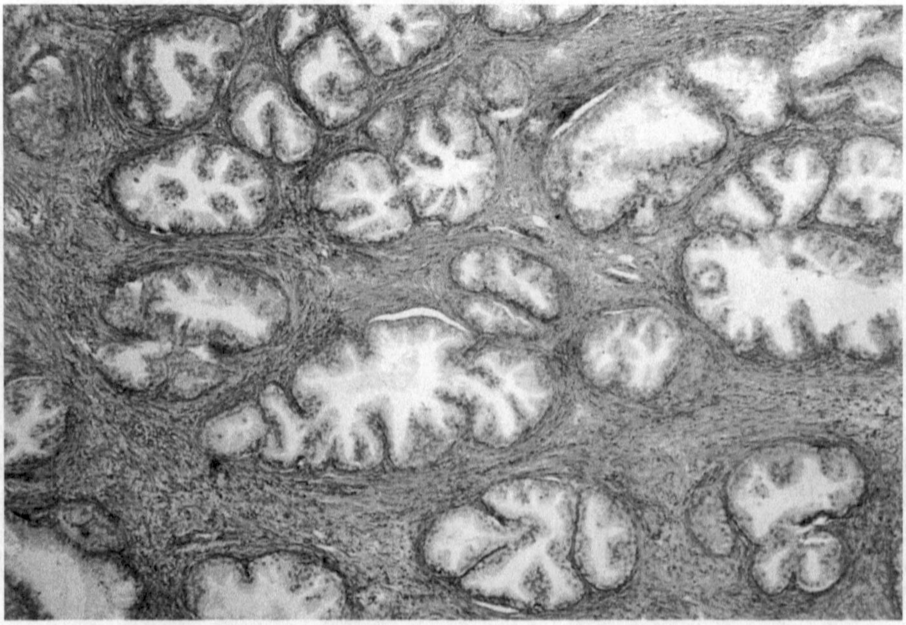

Fig. 1 Human BPH: stromal stimulation after tamoxifen treatment.

To neutralize estrogens *antiestrogens* and *aromatase inhibitors* offer themselves as therapeutic possibilities. Attempts of treatment with the antiestrogen tamoxifen in a dose of 80 mg/d proved unsuccessful in our hands [10]. Tamoxifen administration for 4 weeks before prostatectomy caused stromal stimulation as can be seen in figure 1. Stereological light microscopy analysis of these BPH samples shows a relative enlargement of the smooth muscle cell compartment in tamoxifen treated patients (fig. 2). This effect can be ascribed to tamoxifen metabolites with estrogenic character. In CPA treated patients the decrease of the acinar parenchyma volume results in a relative but not absolute increase of the stroma which shows regressive changes microscopically.

As male estrogen production occurs mostly by extratesticular aromatisation of androstenedione to estrone and of testosterone to estradiol, it was obvious to check on the aromatase activity in BPH.

In fibroblast cultures Schweikert et al. [6] demonstrated endogenous prostatic aromatase activity. Stone et al. [9] confirmed these results in prostatic specimens. Furthermore, a higher rate of aromatisation in fibroblasts of BPH tissue than in prostatic carcinoma was proven [6]. In contrast to these findings Voigt and Bartsch were unable to detect aromatase activity in BPH [13].

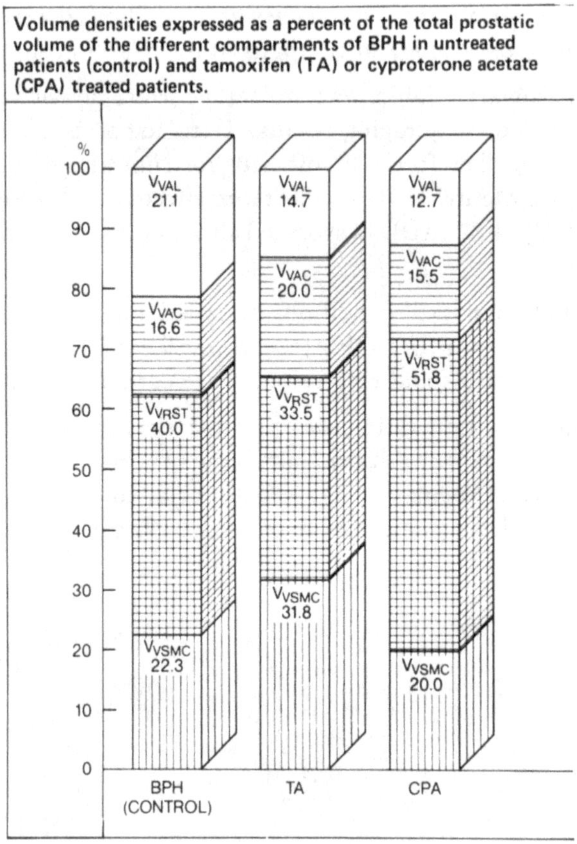

Fig. 2 Human BPH: stereological analysis after tamoxifen and cyproterone acetate treatment.

Aromatase inhibitors and BPH – experimental and clinical results

In a clinical pilot study on BPH and aromatase inhibitors in 1983 we used testolactone [7, 12]. At this time testolactone was the only aromatase inhibitor available for clinical use. In later experimental studies we used 4-hydroxyandrostenedione (4-OHADD) and the newly developed aromatase inhibitor 1-Methyl-Androsta-1,4-diene-3,7-dione (1-Methyl-ADD).

In the clinical pilot study on 13 BPH patients who needed suprapubic drainage because of chronic infravesical obstruction testolactone 200 mg/d. was administered per os for 6 months. Afterwards, 7 patients (group A) could void spontaneously without residual urine while 6 patients could not (group B). Regarding prostatic volumes measured by transrectal sonometry group A showed a reduction of 26% of the initial volume on average in comparison to 15% in group B.

This pilot study with the aromatase inhibitor testolactone which showed no side effects in any patient provided encouraging results. Testolactone is a relatively weak aromatase inhibitor and therefore not sufficient for clinical use. The new substances 4-OHADD and 1-Methyl-ADD are far more effective and were tested in animal experiments [1, 2]. 4-OHADD was tested in a dog model, 1-Methyl-ADD in a monkey model.

In the *dog experiments* under identical conditions castrated animals in group II received androstenedione, in group III 4-OHADD (20 mg/kg BW) additionally. Group I consisted of intact controls and received only the carrier substance.

The 3 groups showed no significant differences in prostatic weight. Yet histomorphological sections showed marked distinctions some of which are presented in figure 3. The control group exhibits characteristic acini lined with simple columnar epithelium surrounded by thin septae of stromal tissue (fig 3 a). An-

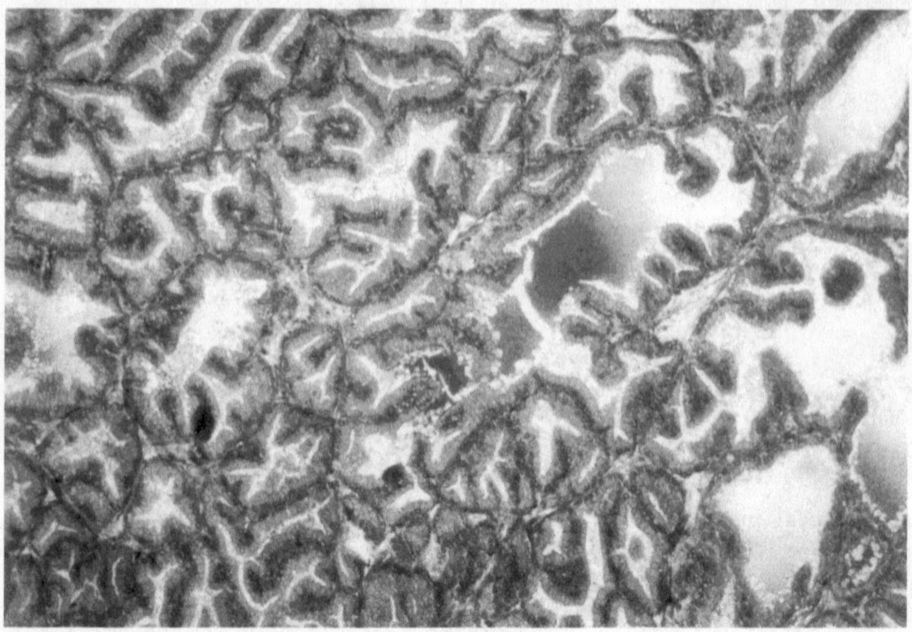

a

Fig. 3 Representative histological prostate sections of the dog experiments:
a) group I: intact control
b) group II: stromal stimulation after androstenedione treatment
c) group III: blockage of stromal stimulation after treatment with androstenedione + 4-OHADD.

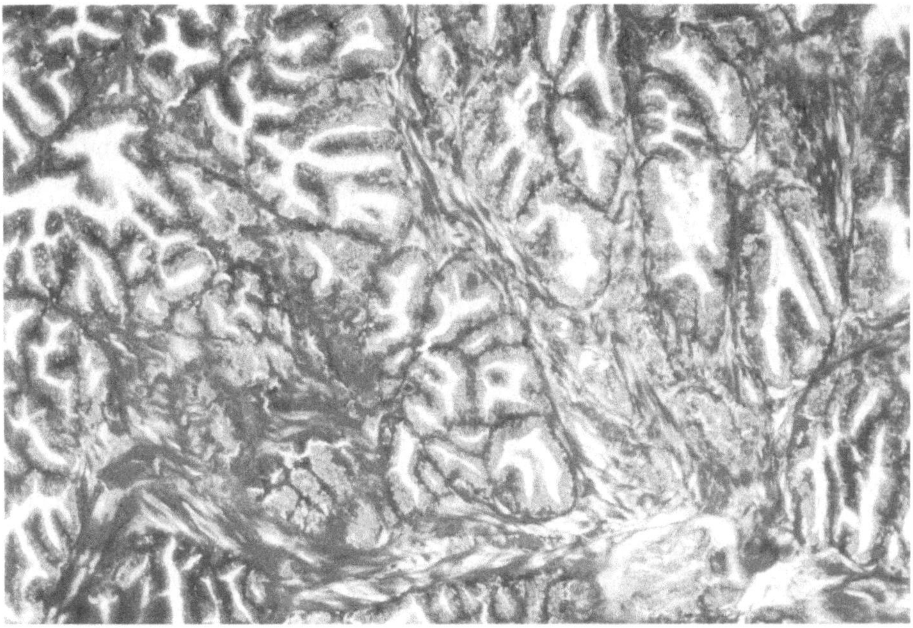

b

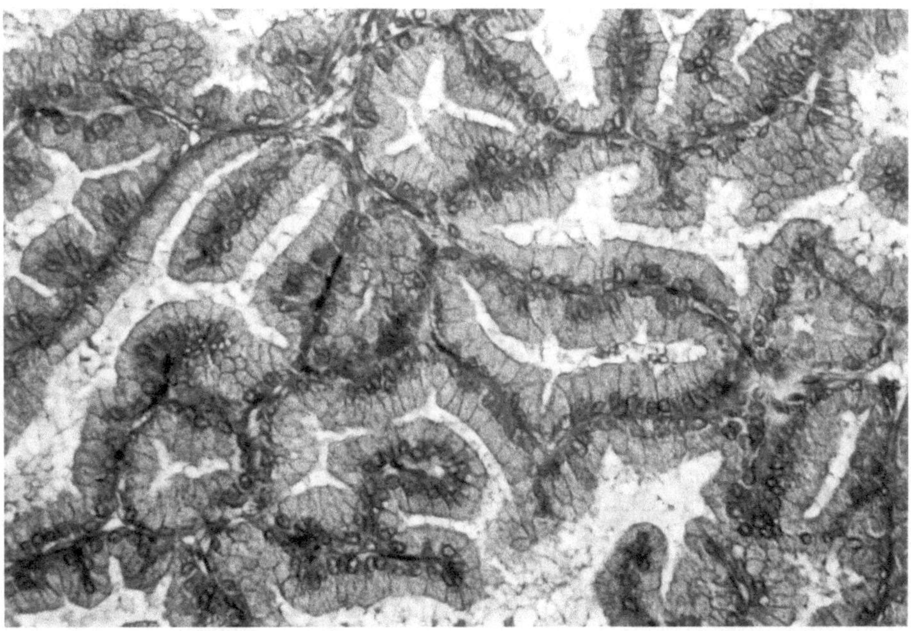

c

drostenedione administration in group II results in regional differences of acinar epithelium. In the peripheral region the morphological appearance of acini is normal whereas activation of the fibromuscular tissue is obvious. This is more pronounced in the intermediate portion of the gland. In the central region cystically enlarged acini with cuboidal epithelium and increased amount of stimulated stroma is seen. Stromal stimulation is to be interpreted as an estrogen effect of the aromatizable androstenedione whereas the intact structure and function of the acinar epithelium is androgen dependent (fig. 3 b). In group III dogs which were treated with androstenedione and the aromatase inhibitor 4-OHADD stromal stimulation is not demonstrable (fig. 3 c).

Quantifying the descriptive morphological findings by light-microscopic stereological analysis the 3 groups show no significant differences regarding acinar parenchyma (fig. 4 a). A slight increase of SMC volume in group II and residual stroma in group III is to be mentioned. Regarding the absolute stromal volumes there is an increase of residual stroma in groups II and III to about double size.

Figure 4 b gives the absolute SMC volumes. The most impressive result is the increase of SMC after androstenedione treatment in group II and the decrease in group III after additional administration of 4-OHAD.

The morphological analysis of these experimental results in the dog model allows the conclusion that estrogen related stimulation of SMC can be neutralized by aromatase inhibitors.

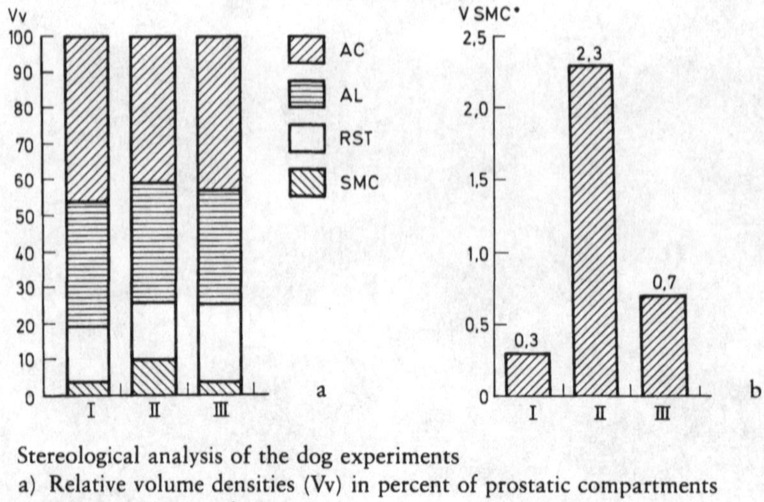

Fig. 4 Stereological analysis of the dog experiments
a) Relative volume densities (Vv) in percent of prostatic compartments
AC: acinar parenchyma
AL: acinar lumina
RST: residual stroma
SMC: smooth muscle cell
b) Absolute volumes (g) of the smooth muscle cell compartment (v SM)

In the *monkey experiments* using cynomolgi the new aromatase inhibitor 1-Methyl-ADD was administered. Again the animals were divided into 3 groups, group I serving as intact controls, group II receiving androstenedione (5 mg/kg BW), and group III receiving androstenedione and 1-Methyl-ADD (30 mg/kg BW) for 3 months.

We would like to point at the important results of this study in spotlight fashion using histological sections in this context. A coronal section of the prostate of the cynomolgus monkey showing the peripheral zone, the ejaculatory ducts and the urethra is shown in figure 5 a.

Peripheral and central zones both consist of epithelial and stromal elements. In the central zone the acinar cells are higher than in the peripheral zone. In both regions the typical stromal tissue can be found. In comparison to the dog there is a higher part of stromal volume in control animals.

As the most impressive result of androstenedione administration a marked stimulation of interacinar tissue occured. This stimulation was more pronounced in the central region than in the periphery. Figure 5 b demonstrates stromal stimulation.

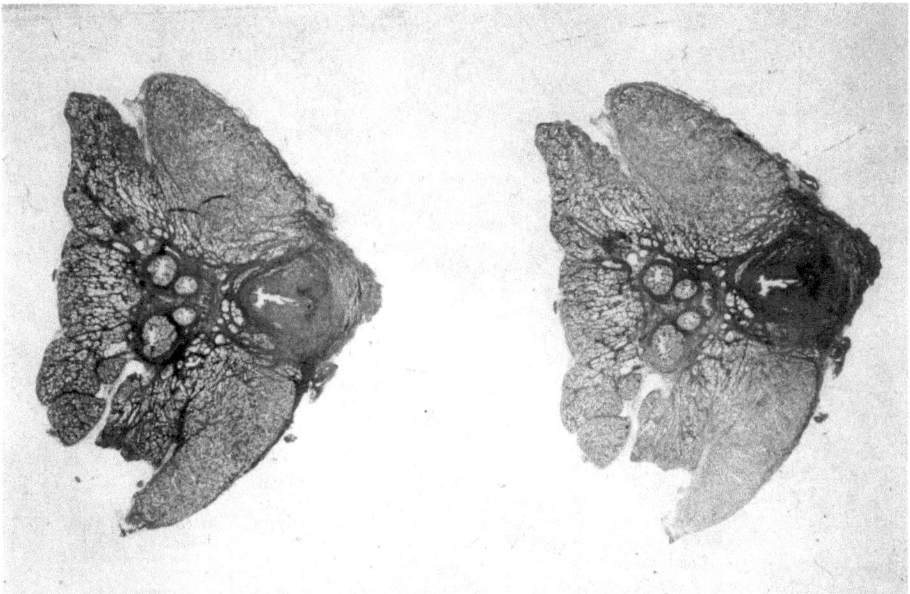

Fig. 5 Representative histological prostate sections of the monkey (cynomolgus) experiments

Fig. 5a) coronal section of the normal prostate (group I)

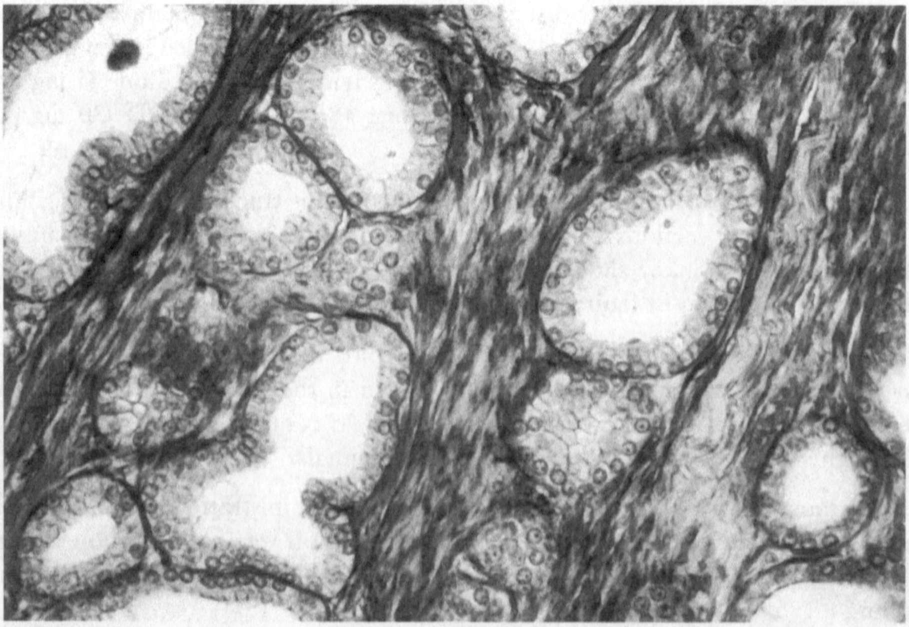

Fig. 5b) stromal stimulation in group II – monkeys after androstenedione treatment

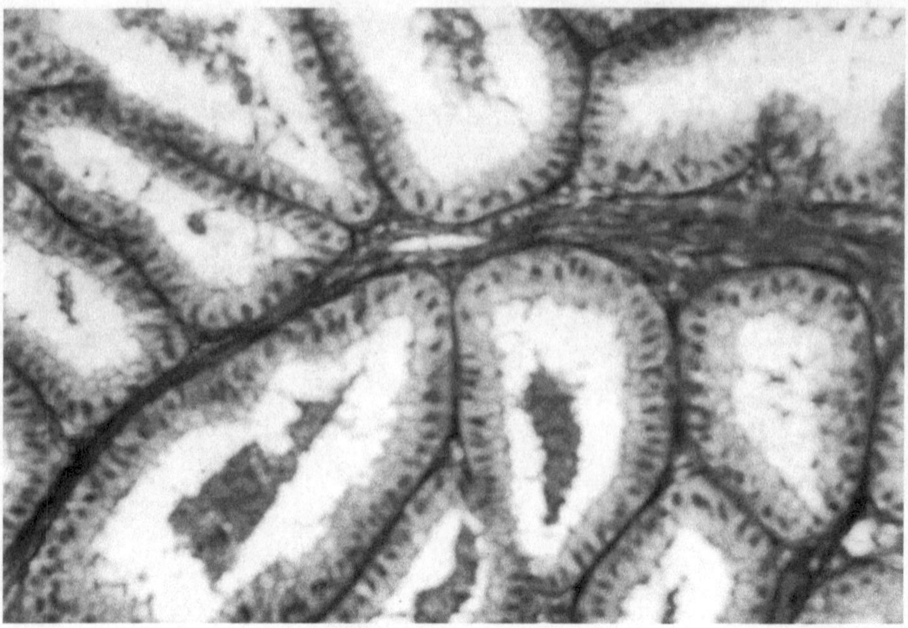

Fig. 5c) antagonisation of stromal stimulation after treatment with androstenedione and 1-Methyl-ADD (group III)

Stromal stimulation was antagonized if the aromatase inhibitor 1-Methyl-ADD was administered simultaneously with androstenedione. In this group stromal stimulation could be demonstrated, but its morphological appearance is comparable to the control group. This neutralizing effect could be seen in all group III animals.

So in animal experiments stromal proliferation as is typical for human BPH can be inhibited at least partially by the new aromatase inhibitor 1-Methyl-ADD.

The relative volumes measured stereologically support the descriptive findings: a rise in absolute stromal volume occurs after androstenedione administration. After androstenedione plus 1-Methyl-ADD the stromal volume is reduced to values comparable to untreated controls (fig. 6).

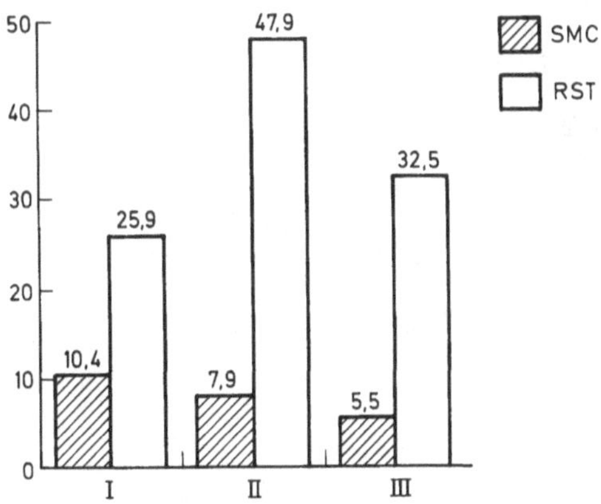

Fig. 6 Relative stromal prostatic volume densities (Vv) in percent in the monkey experiments
group I: intact control
group II: treatment with androstenedione
group III: treatment with androstenedione plus 1-Methyl-ADD

So far there are only clinical data regarding the influence of 1-Methyl-ADD on steroid serum concentrations. In a clinical study the influence of 1-Methyl-ADD on the serum concentrations of testosterone, DHT, E_1 and E_2 one week preoperatively was investigated.

Figure 7 shows the significant decrease of E_1 and E_2 during the application for one week. Discontinuing 1-Methyl-ADD will reverse this effect back to normal. Testosterone and DHT were not affected in this short time study.

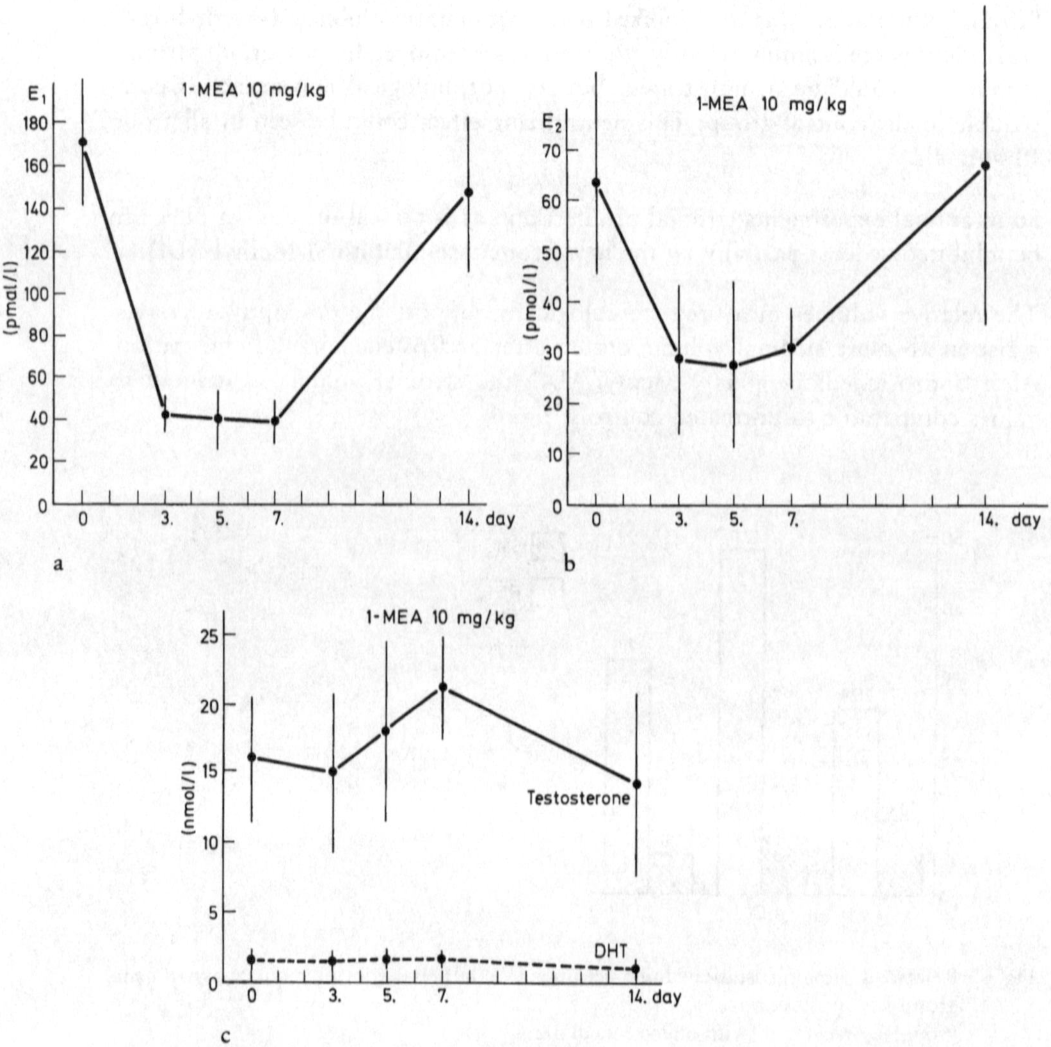

Fig. 7 Serum concentrations of E_1 (fig. 7 a), E_2 (fig. 7 b) and testosterone and DHT (fig. 7 c) in patients treated with 1-Methyl-ADD for 7 days

Conclusion

The results of the experimental studies and the first clinical applications lead to the following conclusions about aromatase inhibitors and BPH:

1. Experimental results in dogs and monkeys demonstrate that aromatase inhibitors are able to reduce estrogen related stromal stimulation in BPH.

2. Low dose testolactone treatment in 13 patients with BPH resulted in a decrease of BPH volume.
3. After treatment of 20 patients with 1-Methyl-ADD for one week a significant decrease of E_1 and E_2 was demonstrable.
4. With the aromatase inhibitor 1-Methyl-ADD a new substance is available which could be the basis for an attractive concept for pharmacological treatment of human BPH. But the pill as an alternative to surgical treatment of BPH can not yet be advocated despite these beginnings.

References

[1] Habenicht, U. F., K. Schwarz, H. U. Schweikert et al.: Development of a Model for the Induction of Estrogen-Related Prostatic Hyperplasia in the Dog and its Response to the Aromatase Inhibitor 4-Hydroxy-4-Androstene-3,17-Dione: Preliminary Results. The Prostate *8* (1986) 181–194.

[2] Habenicht, U. F., K. Schwarz, F. Neumann et al.: Induction of Estrogen-Related Hyperplastic Changes in the Prostate of the Cynomolgus Monkey (Macaca fascicularis) by Androstenedione and its Antagonization by the Aromatase Inhibitor 1-Methyl-Androsta-1,4-Diene-3,17-Dione. The Prostate *11* (1987) 313–326.

[3] Karr, J. P., G. P. Murphy: Cellular growth and hormone receptor. In: F. Hinman, Jr. (ed.): Benign Prostatic Hypertrophy, pp. 193–214. Springer-Verlag, New York 1983.

[4] Kozak, I., W. Bartsch, M. Krieg et al.: Nuclei of stroma: site of highest estrogen concentration in human benign prostatic hyperplasia. The Prostate *3* (1982) 433–438.

[5] Krieg, M., G. Kloetzl, J. Kaufmann et al.: Stroma of benign prostatic hyperplasia: preferential tissue for androgen metabolism and oestrogen binding. Acta endocr., Copenh. *96* (1981) 422–432.

[6] Schweikert, H. U.: Conversion of androstenedione to estrone in human fibroblasts cultured from prostate, genital and nongenital skin. Horm. Metab. Res. *11* (1979) 635–640.

[7] Schweikert, H. U., U. W. Tunn: Effects of the aromatase inhibitor testolactone on human benign prostatic hyperplasia. Steroids 1988 (In press).

[8] Schweikert, H. U., U. W. Tunn: Periphere Östrogenbildung aus Androgenen beim Mann. Akt. Urol. *16* (1985) 64–68.

[9] Stone, N. N., W. R. Fair, J. Fischman: Estrogen formation in human prostatic tissue from patients with and without benign prostatic hyperplasia. The Prostate *4* (1986) 311–318.

[10] Tunn, U. W., T. Senge, H. Schulze et al.: Antihormone und menschliche benigne Prostatahyperplasie. In: K. Bandhauer, H. Toggenburg, H. W. Bauer (eds): Die Prostatahyperplasie, pp. 143–151. W. Zuckschwerdt Verlag, München 1982.

[11] Tunn, U. W., H. U. Schweikert: Endokrinologische Aspekte der Pathogenese der benignen Prostatahyperplasie. In: B. Helpap, T. Senge, W. Vahlensieck (eds): Prostatahyperplasie, pp. 67–86. pmi Verlag, Frankfurt 1983.

[12] Tunn, U. W., P. Kaivers, H. U. Schweikert: Conservative treatment of human benign prostatic hyperplasia. In: N. Bruchovsky, A. Chapdelaine, F. Neumann (eds): Regulation of androgen action, pp. 87–90. Congressdruck R. Brückner, Berlin 1985.

[13] Voigt, K. D., W. Bartsch: Intratissular androgens in benign prostatic hyperplasia and prostatic cancer. J. Steroid Biochem. 25 (1986) 749–757.

Closing remarks

H. Frohmüller

Dear Colleagues and Friends,

We have already exceeded the time that was allocated for our symposium, so I will keep my remarks brief.

I am certain that all of you will agree with me that this was an excellent symposium. It dealt with a subject in which I have had a particular interest ever since I started my training in Urology at the Mayo Clinic, back in 1958. On the one hand it was interesting to see that some of the aspects concerning benign prostatic hyperplasia have hardly undergone any change during these past thirty years, whereas on the other hand intensive research has come up to new ideas in the understanding of BPH especially with regard to its etiology and, basing upon these developments, furthering possibilities for different types of management in the future. This proves a saying by Dr. Charles Mayo "today the only thing that is permanent is change". Or – being a pupil of the Mayo Clinic – to quote Dr. Charlie's brother, Dr. William Mayo: "The glory of medicine is that it is constantly moving forward, that there is always more to learn".

I do not intend to repeat and to re-run this meeting, but I certainly want to thank all of you who participated here. I congratulate the speakers on the outstanding qualities of their contributions. We all appreciated the lively discussions. In particular I thank those of you who have come from abroad and even from overseas. I take special delight in the fact that Dr. David C. Utz, the former Chairman of the Department of Urology at my second Alma Mater, the Mayo Clinic, has come across the ocean to participate at this meeting. I take it as a sign of the uninterrupted close ties since my fellowship at this great institution to which I owe so much in my career.

As the invitation for this Symposium indicated, it was arranged on the occasion of my 60th birthday. Therefore, I should like to express my sincere gratitude to the organizers of the meeting, namely to Prof. Rolf Ackermann, Düsseldorf, and Prof. Fritz Schröder, Rotterdam. Both worked with me at our Department of Urology in Würzburg for quite a number of years, and I am proud to see their accomplishments at their present institutions. I'd like to state, however, that it was certainly not *my* intention to celebrate my birthday with a symposium. But before any information reached me, the program had been set up already and the speakers had been invited. Thus, I was simply confronted with the facts. But inspite of this surprise I must admit that I thoroughly enjoyed our symposium.

I finally want so say a vote of thanks to those members of my department who were responsible for working out the details of our meeting. They performed this task with that kind of meticulous care which I favour so much in our daily endeavours. In these thanks are included my secretary, Mrs. Burkard, who probably carried the largest load, and the other secretaries, as well as Drs. Wirth, Heckl, Grups and other members of the resident staff.

Last but not least I thank all the sponsoring companies mentioned in the program for their support of this symposium. Thank you all once again.

Contributors

Ackermann, R., M. D., Professor and Chairman, Department of Urology, University of Düsseldorf, Medical School, Moorenstr. 5, D-4000 Düsseldorf, F. R. Germany

Andersen, J. T., M. D., Ph. D., Chief Urologist, Department of Urology, Hvidovre Hospital, Kettegaard Alle 30, DK-2650 Hvidovre, Denmark

Aumüller, G., M. D., Professor and Chairman, Department of Anatomy and Cell Biology, Philipps University, D-3550 Marburg-Lahn, F. R. Germany

Bandhauer, K., M. D., Professor and Chairman, Department of Urology, Kantonsspital, CH-9007 St. Gallen, Switzerland

Bartsch, G., M. D., Professor and Chairman, Department of Urology, University of Innsbruck, Anichstr. 35, A-6020 Innsbruck, Austria

Begun, F. P., M. D., Assistant Professor, Department of Urology, The Medical College of Wisconsin, 9200 West Wisconsin Avenue, Milwaukee, Wisconsin 53226, USA

Blom, J. H. M., M. D., Department of Urology, Erasmus University, P. O. Box 1700, N-3000 DR Rotterdam, The Netherlands

Bosch, R. J. L. H., M. D., Department of Urology, Erasmus University, P. O. Box 1700, N-3000 DR Rotterdam, The Netherlands

Brüngger, A., M. D., Department of Pathology, University of Basel, Kantonsspital CH-4030 Basel, Switzerland

Bülow, H., M. D., Professor and Chairman, Department of Urology, Leopoldina-Krankenhaus, Gustav-Adolf-Straße 8, D-8720 Schweinfurt, F. R. Germany

Dreikorn, K., M. D., Professor and Chairman, Department of Urology, Zentralkrankenhaus, St. Jürgen-Str., D-2800 Bremen, F. R. Germany

Hintner, H., M. D., Department of Dermatology, University of Innsbruck, Anichstr. 35, A-6020 Innsbruck, Austria

Isaacs, J. T., M. D., Department of Urology and Oncology Center, Johns Hopkins School of Medicine, Baltimore, Maryland 21205, USA

Jacobs, S. C., M. D., Professor, Department of Urology, The Medical College of Wisconsin, 9200 West Wisconsin Avenue, Milwaukee, Wisconsin 53226, USA

Jensen, K. M.-E., M. D., Chief Urologist, Department of Urology, Hvidovre Hospital, Kettegaard Alle 30, DK-2650 Hvidovre, Denmark

Lawson, R. K., M. D., Professor and Chairman, Department of Urology, The Medical College of Wisconsin, 9200 West Wisconsin Avenue, Milwaukee, Wisconsin 53226, USA

Mawhinney, M. G., M. D., Ph. D., Professor of Urology and Pharmacology/Toxicology, Departments of Urology and Pharmacology, West Virginia University Medical Center, Morgantown, West Virginia 26506, USA

Richter, R., M. D., Department of Urology, Zentralkrankenhaus, St. Jürgen-Str., D-2800 Bremen, F. R. Germany

Rohr, H. P., M. D., Department of Pathology, University of Basel, Kantonsspital, CH-4030 Basel, Switzerland

Romijn, J. C., Ph. D., Department of Urology, Erasmus University, P. O. Box 1738, N-3000 DR Rotterdam, The Netherlands

Schröder, F. H., M. D., Professor and Chairman, Department of Urology, Erasmus University Rotterdam, P. O. Box 1700, N-3000 DR Rotterdam, The Netherlands

Schweikert, H. U., M. D., Professor, Department of Internal Medicine, University of Bonn, Wilhelmstr. 35 – 37, D-5300 Bonn, F. R. G.

Di Silverio, F., M. D., Professor and Chairman, Department of Urology, University "La Sapienza", I-Rome, Italy

Story, M. T., Ph. D., Department of Urology, The Medical College of Wisconsin, 9200 West Wisconsin Avenue, Milwaukee, Wisconsin 53226, USA

Tenaglia, R., M. D., Professor and Chairman, Department of Urology, University "G. D'Annunzio", Via A. Vignani, I-66100 Chieti, Italy

Tunn, U. W., M. D., Professor and Chairman, Department of Urology, Städtische Kliniken, Postfach 10 19 64, D-6050 Offenbach, F. R. Germany

Utz, D. C., M. D., Professor and Chairman, Department of Urology, Mayo-Clinic, 200 1st Street, Rochester, Minnesota 55905, USA

FSC
www.fsc.org
MIX
Papier | Fördert
gute Waldnutzung
FSC® C083411

Zeitfracht Medien GmbH
Ferdinand-Jühlke-Straße 7
99095 Erfurt, Deutschland
produktsicherheit@kolibri360.de